DIABETES IN NATIVE CHICAGO

DIABETES IN NATIVE CHICAGO

An Ethnography of Identity, Community, and Care

MARGARET POLLAK

University of Nebraska Press

LINCOLN

Portions of chapter 1 first appeared in "Reflections on Urban Migration," *American Indian Culture and Research Journal* 40, no. 3 (2016): 85–102. Portions of chapter 6 first appeared in "Care in the Context of a Chronic Epidemic: Caring for Diabetes in Chicago's Native Community," *Medical Anthropology Quarterly* 32, no. 2 (2018): 196–213.

Library of Congress Cataloging-in-Publication Data
Names: Pollak, Margaret, author.
Title: Diabetes in Native Chicago: an ethnography of identity, community, and care / Margaret Pollak.
Description: Lincoln: University of Nebraska Press, 2021. | Includes bibliographical references and index.
Identifiers: LCCN 2021008004
ISBN 9781496212061 (hardback)
ISBN 9781496228482 (epub)
ISBN 9781496228499 (pdf)
Subjects: LCSH: Diabetes. | Diabetes—Illinois. | Diabetes—Treatment—Illinois—Chicago. | Indians of North America—Diseases—Illinois—Chicago. | Indians of North American—Health and hygiene.
Classification: LCC RA645.D5 P64 2021
DDC 362.1964/6200977311—dc23
LC record available at https://lccn.loc.gov/2021008004

Set in Arno Pro by Laura Buis.

CONTENTS

TABLES

ACKNOWLEDGMENTS

I am deeply indebted to Chicago's Native community. The American Indian Center of Chicago served as my base site over the course of the decade during which this work developed. I not only received support and encouragement from community members I encountered at the center but also developed a deeper understanding of past and contemporary urban Indigenous American life through my conversations with people there. I am grateful for the experiences Chicago's Native community has shared with me over the course of this research.

The process of writing this book was also supported by peer and faculty mentors in university settings along the way, whom I acknowledge chronologically here. At Cornell College Alfrieta Parks Monagan sparked in me an interest in anthropology that has never faded. In my first year of graduate school, Anthony Webster put me in touch with the executive director of American Indian Center, which got the ball rolling on this work, for which I am very grateful. I view my master's thesis work at Southern Illinois University as being invaluably formative for me as a scholar, and I thank my mentors from that time, Roberto Barrios, Anthony Webster, David Sutton, Janet Fuller, and Jonathan Hill. When I moved to the University of Wisconsin to begin work on a PhD, I was fortunate to find a mentor in Claire

Wendland. I am sincerely grateful for her advice and encouragement throughout my graduate and early professional career. I further appreciate the insights of my committee members and professors at the University of Wisconsin, Maria Lepowsky, Larry Nesper, Linda Hogle, Shannon Sparks, Alexandra Adams, Kirin Narayan, Kenneth George, Katherine Bowie, and Daniel Kleinman, and my peers at the same university who opened my mind to new perspectives on the field, on fieldwork, and on life more generally: Maria Frias, Wang Bo, Kiersten Warning, Christina Cappy, Chisato Fukuda, and Rachael Goodman. I am further grateful for the support I enjoyed as I began editing my dissertation into a book at both Northwestern University and Indiana University–Northwest. Bill Leonard, Kim Rapp, Devora Greenspan, Noelle Sullivan, Beatriz Oralia Reyes, Kelly Wisecup, Kevin McElmurry, Tanice Foltz, Charles Gallmeier, Jack Bloom, and Jonathyne Briggs have all played a role in my development in these early years of my career.

This research was made possible through the generous support of the National Science Foundation Cultural Anthropology Program (award number BCS-1226577), the Robert Wood Johnson Health and Society Scholars Program (award number 053574), the American Philosophical Society, and the University of Wisconsin's Graduate School, Holtz Center for Science and Technology Studies, and Anthropology Department. Additionally, I am thankful to Helen Murtaugh for providing me with a home in Chicago during the early stages of this study.

Finally, my family and friends have supported me throughout the entirety of this project. I would like to thank my parents, Dennis and Janice Collier, for their unwavering support; my cohort of undergraduate friends Alexa Sedlacek, Kacie Flaherty, and Stephanie Penn for their encouragement; and Micah Pollak for his support and partnership.

Any errors within the following pages are mine alone.

INTRODUCTION

Holly and I reclined on armrests on opposite sides of the turquoise velvet couch in the Little One's room at the American Indian Center of Chicago.[1] The age and disrepair of the former Masonic temple is felt through its inability to equally distribute and retain heat on this cold January day. Holly's awareness of the uneven heating pattern, evident in her choice of wearing multiple layers—a gray and turquoise patterned shirt, topped with a draping black cardigan sweater—is a testament to her intimate knowledge of this center. Holly, a forty-four-year-old Apache/Sioux woman, was raised in Chicago by parents who both developed diabetes later in life. In our conversation, Holly noted that Natives have higher rates of diabetes than other ethnic populations:

> HOLLY: One of the things that I think of in our diets that our bodies aren't used to as Native people is that the settlers brought, the government brought, gave us white products—the salt, the sugar, the flour, dairy, all those things were things our bodies weren't used to, and they each took a toll and, you know some of those things together or separate, however you want to say it, came in the form of bringing diabetes . . . I think the bodies aren't able to process it. I think that Native people are used to very natural diets where they ate off the land, they ate grains, they drank teas from the earth. Everything was very simple and very pure.

Holly's explanation highlights several conceptions about diabetes shared commonly by members of Chicago's Native community: first, that Native people did not encounter diseases like diabetes prior to contact with settler communities; second, that Indigenous North Americans share a similar physiology that predisposes them to developing diabetes; and third, that the precolonial diet of Indigenous Americans was one of purity before being interrupted and contaminated by contact with white settlers. In the Columbian Exchange, European bodies brought diseases that Native bodies were not prepared to combat. Decades of early contact and the related social disruptions created a context wherein Native bodies were particularly susceptible to these new diseases, including smallpox, typhus, and measles.[2] Today's epidemics in Native communities—diabetes, obesity, alcoholism, depression, and intergenerational trauma—are thought of by many urban Natives in similar terms; that is, it is perceived that these conditions arrived as a result of prolonged contact with European bodies and lifeways and are devastating to Indigenous American communities.

This book argues that the relationship between human culture and human biology is a reciprocal one, in which colonial history has produced the diabetes epidemic in Native populations, which is itself being incorporated into contemporary discussions of ethnic identity in Native Chicago, where a vulnerability to the development of the condition is described as a distinctly Native trait. In doing so, this text travels along related tributaries exploring Native identity, urban migration, urban Native life, and acts of care within Chicago's Native community.

Background

Indigenous Americans have some of the highest rates of diabetes in the world, and they are disproportionately affected by the secondary complications of the disease when compared with other ethnic populations in the United States of America.[3] While prior to World War II the occurrence of diabetes was rare among Indigenous Americans, over the past sixty-five years rates have risen dramatically.[4] Through a study of Indian Health Service records, the Centers for Disease Control and Prevention (CDC) have found that 14.7 percent of the adult Indigenous population in the United States have been diagnosed with diabetes; this rate varies greatly by tribe, with Alaska Natives reporting 5.5 percent of the population with diabetes and the Akimel O'odham of the Gila River Reservation (also known as the Pima Indians) reporting 50 percent of their thirty-five-year-old and older population as diabetic.[5] Much of the data collected by the CDC and other researchers, however, is gathered from reservation clinics. The focus of data collection on reservations continues today despite nearly 80 percent of people of Native ancestry living outside of reservation areas.[6] Though there are less data available on the diagnosis rates in urban settings, the disease is prevalent among urban Native populations in those metropolitan areas where studies have been completed; 19.8 percent of those over the age of forty-five in Los Angeles in 1992 and 21 percent of those over the age of fifty in Seattle in 2004 had been diagnosed with the disease.[7]

This book focuses on diabetes care and understandings in an urban Native population in Chicago, Illinois. No published rates of diabetes for this population exist, and the feasibility of accurately estimating rates in the city is complicated by the fact that Chicago Natives utilize a wide variety of health-care providers both in the city and on reservations both near and far. Still, we know that rates of diabetes are high. In one interview, a participant stated, "All the people that I know that are Native American have it." Moreover, the ubiquity of the disease in the community influences diagnosis expectations, care practices, and some discussions of indigeneity in the city space.

Native Chicago

Chicago is home to the eighth largest Indigenous American population. The American Indian Center of Chicago estimates that the greater Chicagoland area is currently home to sixty-five thousand Indigenous Americans representing more than one hundred

Native Nations from across the United States and Canada.[8] Members of Chicago's Native community refer to themselves individually and as a community using a variety of terms—Indian, American Indian, Native, Native American, Indigenous, NDN, and most often by individual tribal affiliation. Herein I refer to members of this community as Natives, Indigenous Americans, and often by tribal affiliation when speaking of an individual to mirror the language of the community. I use a capital N in "Native" to mark the difference between individuals whose ancestors were indigenous to the Americas and those who were born in the United States but whose ancestors came to this land within the past few hundred years.

Researching Diabetes in Native Chicago

This text is based upon ethnographic research that I began in May 2007 at the American Indian Center of Chicago. As the staff meeting at the center concluded on my first day of research, Laura suggested I head over to Tribal Hall to see if I can assist with preparations for the elder lunch. At the time, Laura was the director of the center's wellness program and one of my first contacts in Chicago. I made my way from the meeting in the Little One's room to Diane Maney Tribal Hall, passing through the front reception area where a sign hanging over the receptionist's window informed guests, "You're on Indian Land." Tribal Hall was prepared for the arrival of community members for one of the week's two elder lunches. In the center of the hall, six tables stood in two rows of three. The long and narrow tables, with thin white plastic covers, were surrounded by chairs upholstered in thick burnt-orange fabric stained by years of use. As we served the meal an hour later, I noted the necessities that each table provided for the diners: a bowl filled with red and black salt and pepper packets, a Styrofoam cup with either a creamy white ranch or a syrupy magenta raspberry salad dressing, and a second bowl containing tiny brown tubs of Country Crock brand margarine.

Looking around for someone to give me a task, I noted the north side of the hall, where three tables stood beneath an expansive mural.

Painted by a community artist, this mural depicted three women, each with long dark hair and heavy mustard yellow dresses that cover their arms and reach their ankles; they stand behind a large shallow azure bowl holding the three sisters of Indigenous American diets—corn, beans, and squash. One of the sisters holds the leafy stem of the climbing beans as her eyes meet with the viewer's; the two other sisters are turned in toward one another, looking at something within their own landscape, beyond the sight of the observer.

Upon hearing the sudden clanking of a metal spoon being tapped against a stainless-steel pot, I peered into the doorway to the left of this mural and saw two women inside the kitchen preparing for the twenty-eight diners who would arrive later that day. As I drew nearer to the door, the spiced aroma of beef marinara with onions and green peppers simmering over a gas-lit stove intensified. The women were preparing a tray of individual iceberg lettuce salads. I entered the kitchen to introduce myself and offer help. The women introduced themselves as regular volunteers at the center's lunches and instructed me to pull my hair back and wash my hands before helping with anything. I helped with menial tasks, like ensuring the water container was full and washing dishes, while the regular volunteers made the lunch—a salad with carrots, broccoli, and croutons, a plate of spaghetti with the meat and pepper marinara and a slice of whole wheat sandwich bread, finished with a thin slice of sweet potato pie topped with pecans for dessert. I later learned that to work alongside the regular staff and volunteers in the center's kitchen, one must first prove one's competence through the successful completion of menial work.

This senior meal at the center foreshadowed in its very mundaneness some of the important symbolic and pragmatic issues in contemporary urban Native diabetes I was to learn about in subsequent years. On this first day of my research in May of 2007—which was the first of four periods of ethnographic fieldwork studying diabetes in Chicago's Native community—I assisted with my first of nearly one hundred meal preparations at the center and began to forge relationships with members of Chicago's Native community. My goal was to document the experience, care, and understanding of the disease from the perspective of people living with diabetes and people providing care for it.

After just one month of research in the summer of 2007, I was elated to receive an invitation to participate in a seminar on diabetes in Chicago's Native community. The seminar took place in the center's wellness department office. Laura, Rebecca (the director of the center's elder program and the only person of Native ancestry in this meeting), Wendy (the center's dietician), Fred (a social work intern), and I sat around Laura's recently cleared desk to discuss a range of topics related to diabetes—prevention, symptoms, diagnosis, education, research, and care. Having not run into any significant resistance to my presence at the center up to this point, I was unprepared for what was to come next.

While discussing how aspects of Native culture and history affect diabetes treatment, trust emerged as a prominent issue. Wendy had been speaking about the frequent research surveys brought into elder lunches when Rebecca shifted the topic of discussion to the position of outside researchers: "We don't trust people that sit in the corner with notebooks." I immediately realized that though Rebecca's passing statement was directed at no one in particular, I was implicated in the comment. As a novice anthropologist I had kept my pink and green checkered notebook with me at all times to jot down observations and thoughts during the past month; even at the very moment of Rebecca's remark, I was jotting down Wendy's statement about how the community had been "surveyed to death." The seminar continued on as Laura transitioned the conversation toward the types of food offered at the center's events. As I drove home later that afternoon, I began to question the goals and motivations behind my research.

My own personal experiences with diabetes both initiated and deeply influenced my scholarship. I was diagnosed with type 1 diabetes in adolescence and have observed family members caring for type 2 diabetes throughout much of my life. My interest in the eventual topic of my dissertation research was spurred by my curiosity to know how culture and history shape the experience of diabetes. While my own experience with diabetes greatly affected my initial research aims and practices, Rebecca's comment more significantly shaped the way I approached research in the community in the years that followed. After that day I began to familiarize myself with Indigenous critiques of research in their communities. Vine Deloria Jr.'s chapter on anthropologists in *Custer Died for Your Sins* was an eye-opening introduction that led me to the work of Cecil King, Devon Abbott Mihesuah, Linda Tuhiwai Smith, each informing my understandings of what responsibilities I have as an ethnographer to those who share their experiences with me.[9] In addition to the perspectives of scholars on decolonizing methodologies, in later phases of research I listened to local community voices on research practices. While in Chicago I not only conducted research but also volunteered at the American Indian Center of Chicago whenever I was not actively engaged in research work; I have also returned to present my findings at community conferences.

This book is based on a total of twenty-five months of ethnographic research conducted with Chicago's Indigenous population between 2007 and 2017. I began with interviews and observations at the American Indian Center and expanded from there through contacts made at the center. Participants for this study were recruited using the snowball method of sampling. First working with the wellness department of the American Indian Center, I met several medical practitioners, diabetes patients, and caregivers. Those first interviewees introduced me to other research participants. In total I completed 124 interviews with 97 participants (see appendix 1). Interviewees identified themselves as citizens of Indigenous American Nations from across the United States and Canada (see appendix 1). Beginning in 2010 grant funding provided monies to compensate interviewees twenty dollars for their time and travel to the interview site. Prior to 2010 I did not compensate participants.

The material collected through interviews was complemented by observational material. In Chicago I observed the day-to-day running of the center, its programs, and larger community events, including powwows, holiday celebrations, and educational forums. Informal conversations that emerged in the day-to-day interactions at the center and in the community also informed this work. Conversations with community members about diabetes and other health concerns, including cancer, heart disease, and intergenerational trauma, and about the community and state of the center arose in daily interactions—while taking a lunch break during the Thursday food pantry, when someone stopped by for a chat while I sat at the reception desk, as we prepared the elder lunch on Wednesdays, or in cars while stuck in Chicago traffic.[10] These discussions about life in Chicago, Native health, the history of the community, and Native history have supplemented my understandings gained through formal interviews. In November of 2015 I collected dietary surveys at a community event held at the center. Fifty-three community members completed an eleven-page survey with questions about their demographic information, their general health and health care choices, and their typical eating habits.

In addition to gathering data through observations, informal conversations, interviews, and surveys, I also collected print documents and studied archived materials. I collected diabetes-related literature from local community centers, pharmacies, and medical centers visited by community members. I took notes on whom these pamphlets and materials were intended for, the meanings and ideologies communicated, and how communication is accomplished through text. I also completed archival research at the Newberry Library in Chicago, focusing on the history of Chicago's Native community and the federally run Urban Indian Relocation Program. At the library I sought out documents on the relocation program, an oral history pilot project on Chicago's Native community from the 1980s, records from Native organizations in the city, and the documents of other researchers, including those of Virgil Vogel, David R. M. Beck, and Elaine M. Neils, on Native life and history. These documents offer additional context to the story told in this book.

The aim of this study was to document the experience, care, and understanding of diabetes. My lived experience as a diabetic—particularly experiencing cases of high and low blood glucose levels, being acutely aware of my own daily carbohydrate consumption, and working with biomedical providers to develop care routines—influenced the development of the research protocol and my analysis of the data collected. Additionally, my status as a fellow diabetic was also beneficial in the early years of this study when I had fewer contacts in Chicago. During these early years, some community members expressed greater comfort with me as a researcher because I shared some of their experiences in managing diabetes. My presence in this book is ongoing, as much of what I learned was from personal interactions and interviews with individuals.

As noted above, during my months of research I volunteered at the American Indian Center and at other community events in the city. This volunteer work ranged from working at the center's reception desk and food pantry, helping prepare for and clean up after community events, entering data for the center's wellness programs, and cleaning center bathrooms and floors. Volunteering at the center gave me an opportunity to participate in and observe its day-to-day life and further made me visible to community members. Doing so helped me establish relationships with community members, effectively separating myself from the other researchers who arrived at the center to collect data on the community and never return. Within a few years of working in the community, I began presenting my findings at the American Indian Center and have offered my findings to the center and American Indian Health Service of Chicago to be used for grant funding and wellness programming purposes.

Aims

This work is an exploration of the relationship between human culture and human biology. I argue that there is a reciprocal relationship between human culture and biology, wherein history and culture shape modern human health and human health shapes modern culture. I show how colonialism affects bodies and communities through intergenerational trauma, displacement, chronic poverty, and altered foodways. We have long been aware of the devastating toll wrought on the Indigenous populations of the Americas through the Columbian Exchange. As noted in the introduction to this chapter, noncommunicable diseases like diabetes are thought of by some urban Natives in similar terms. While there is a long history of diabetes in human populations extending back three thousand years, the rise of diabetes in the Indigenous populations of the Americas is in fact relatively recent and is attributable to the long-term and continuing impact of colonialism.

I further demonstrate that this ongoing epidemic has influenced Native culture, showing that diabetes, as a disease that Natives are at risk of developing, has been adopted and incorporated into local discussions of Indigenous identity in the urban space. My work shows that Native identity is a complicated, and at times contested issue in Chicago and in Native North America more broadly. As already mentioned, Chicago's Native population is an intertribal one, with citizens representing more than one hundred tribes from the United States and Canada. In local discourse members of the city's Native community articulate a shared Indigenous identity through a shared vulnerability to diabetes that transcends tribal differences. In theorizing how diabetes has been incorporated into these local discourses, I explore the role history and culture play in shaping modern human health and how human health shapes modern culture.

The findings here contribute to the vast scholarship on the Indigenous American diabetes epidemic and move it in a new direction. Medical and historical studies of diabetes in Native North Americans trace the high occurrence of the disease to changes in lifestyle (e.g., land restriction and diet) imposed, in many cases violently, upon Indigenous populations by Western colonial forces.[11] In recent decades medical anthropologists have shifted their attention to Native perceptions of diabetes etiology and to the formation of treatment programs based in local health and treatment models.

Scholars in this vein find that the indiscriminate implementation of biomedical treatment programs is unsuccessful in reservation health-care settings.[12] While Indigenous concepts share some commonalities with those of biomedicine, Indigenous models diverge from biomedical models in viewing psychological stress and spiritual wellness as two significant factors in diabetes etiology.[13] The results of this research have led to the development, implementation and further study of diabetes treatment programs incorporating Native cultural practices like talking circles, native games, and traditional foods.[14]

This text contributes to these studies in two ways. First, the majority of existing anthropological work on the Indigenous American diabetes epidemic has been centered on reservation settings. In contrast, this study focuses on the care and experience of diabetes in an urban setting, where the majority of Indigenous Americans live today. Second, previous studies focus on the causes of diabetes and the challenges of its care in these populations. I approach the study of diabetes in Native communities from a new vantage point, focusing on the influence the epidemic has on contemporary discussions of Indigenous identity.

Chapter Organization

This book is made up of eight sections, including this introduction, six chapters covering the main findings, and a brief conclusion.

In chapter 1 I introduce readers to Chicago's Native population. This chapter first traces the history of the relationship between Indigenous American Nations and the settler community before examining the history of the Urban Indian Relocation Program. While the Indigenous peoples of North America have built and lived in urban areas for millennia, in the years following World War II, with pressure from Urban Indian Relocation and Termination Programs, Natives moved to cities in greater numbers than they had in the centuries before the war.[15] Between 1952 and 1972, one hundred thousand Natives relocated to cities through the federally established Urban Indian Relocation Program that offered housing and employment support, and many others moved to urban locations on their own. In this chapter I show that the Urban Indian Relocation Program was one piece of a larger part of history that aimed at assimilating Indigenous peoples and reducing federal obligations to Native peoples and nations during the mid-twentieth century. In the latter half of this chapter, I put these aims of assimilation in dialogue with elders' and second generation relocatees' reflections upon why they and their families migrated to cities like Chicago, showing that many of the people who moved to Chicago chose to do so in search of opportunities that they could not find on the reservation.

In chapter 2 I describe contemporary Native Chicago. Research on urban Indigenous life focuses largely on the processes and effects of relocation, the maintenance of Native identity in the city, and the development of intertribal movements.[16] I build upon this scholarship by exploring Native identity and community in Chicago. This second chapter explores views of what it means to be Native in an urban context by focusing first on local discussions of blood, race, appearance, shared history, language, and performance; in the process, I examine today's understandings of Native identity in contrast to traditional Native views on social difference. In the second half of the chapter, I describe Chicago's contemporary Native community, illustrating that it is made up of interconnected networks that reach beyond the city to reservation spaces.

In chapter 3 I explore the history of diabetes from antiquity to today, illustrating and contrasting past and current medical models for what diabetes is and why people develop the disease. I describe the development of current understandings of diabetes within biomedicine, the form of medicine participants in this study most often encounter in their care for the condition. In the latter half of this chapter, I turn to the American Indian diabetes epidemic. The first recorded case of diabetes in a Native American individual was in 1902; today Natives have some of the highest rates of diabetes in the world. During the decades following World War II, rates of diabetes in Native populations began to climb; I argue that this is the embodiment of a long history of colonialism and forced migration in Native bodies. Previous scholars have argued that diabetes in Native populations can be explained by the commodity food supplies that made up reservation diets.[17] While this argument is true for Natives living on reservations, it ignores the growing population of urban Natives during that same era. Oral history interviews on Native diets in Chicago during the era of Indian Relocation build upon this history for an urban context.

In chapter 4, I describe diabetes in Native Chicago, showing that high rates of diabetes in urban spaces shape local beliefs, practices, and understandings of the condition. Children in the community learn about diabetes at a young age and in relationships of care, in contrast to non-Native populations who typically learn of diabetes later in life and in classroom settings. For Native children, knowledge of the disease and its care grows with age. This fourth chapter also documents the local views about diabetes in terms of fatalism and moralization about diabetes care. Prevalence in the community, in addition to public health media, influences understandings of diabetes risk for Indigenous Americans. In the last section, I describe an emic classification system that defines diabetes on a scale from mild to full-blown to severe. This system is based in local experiences and observations of the disease, and I contrast it with the biomedical or etic model for diabetes.

In chapter 5 I take a step back and look more broadly at local definitions and explanations for diabetes in the community under study. Scholars have found that lay understandings of health and illness are shaped by local medical models and local experiences.[18] Thus, conceptions of diabetes are situated within the experience and care for diabetes in Native Chicago and local discourses of diabetes offer a look into local world views on evolution, colonial history, and Native identity. In the first half of the chapter, I show that local diabetes definitions are varied and situated within personal experiences with diabetes. In the second, I document local explanations for diabetes with a focus on explanations for high rates of diabetes in Native populations. Local explanations, I demonstrate, not only offer local understandings of diabetes etiology but also strengthen notions of a shared Native identity in this urban space through discussions of shared history and shared bodies.

In the last chapter, I explore how care for diabetes is performed in Chicago. I argue here that care for diabetes goes far beyond individuals' self-care in this highly affected community. In the first section, I look at biomedical care provider expectations for care before discussing factors that influence the performance of these care practices. In the latter section, I describe when, where, how, and by whom care work is performed, showing that both men and women, along with young children, are involved in the day-to-day care of diabetes in Chicago. I also extend studies of care by looking at how in a community facing epidemic rates of disease, care—as thoughtful actions with diabetes treatment in mind—is enmeshed in the everyday lives of not just those living with the disease, but of those in their lives. Members of Chicago's Native community incorporate not only diabetes care but awareness of other chronic condition needs into their lives, and this care is performed by individuals living with the disease, as well as by their family and friends, and at times on a larger community level. This care work is one way in which ties in Chicago's intertribal community are strengthened.

In the conclusion, I summarize the primary findings of this study and further discuss some suggestions to consider as rates of diabetes continue to climb both nationally and internationally. I present the goals of community members for the well-being of their community in the future, arguing that diabetes care in urban Indigenous communities should be a community-engaged project. Communities know their own needs and desires best, and developing plans and programs for tackling diabetes successfully in this and in any other community facing high rates of disease necessitates working closely with community organizers and extending understandings of health and wellness from a focus on the physiological to the more holistic. By this I mean extending our understandings of health to be more inclusive of not just physical health but of the social circumstances that shape well-being.

DIABETES IN NATIVE CHICAGO

1

The Building of Chicago's Contemporary Indigenous American Population

Sunlight illuminated and warmed the west office space on the first floor of the American Indian Center where Elmer and I met to talk about his life and history in the greater Chicago area. Elmer, a seventy-seven-year-old member of the Bad River Band Chippewa—a group that he took care to remind me was not a rock band—was born during his parents' journey from their northern Wisconsin reservation to the Chicago area in the late 1940s. In our conversation about his early life in Elgin, Illinois, Elmer elaborated on his view of the Urban Indian Relocation Program, which began several years after his family had migrated to the Chicago region:

> ELMER: Now with the Urban Indian Relocation, yes, and that was a disaster, I saw Indians relocated even out in Elgin and just . . . it was such a disaster. And the old grandmother was arrested for shoplifting and her kids . . . these people were uprooted and transplanted without any fertilizer, well, even any ground, just transplanted on the rocks out there and it was a disaster . . . they finally ended up shipping these people back or getting out or bringing them to Chicago where they died. It was almost like their continuation of genocide. Unjust. Unjust.

The Urban Indian Relocation Program that Elmer describes as the United States' continuation of genocide was run by the Bureau of Indian Affairs from the 1950s to 1970s. Discussing it elicits mixed responses from Chicago's Native community members. While the program assisted Natives in moving away from poverty and high unemployment rates found on many reservations during that era, the primary aim of the program was to assimilate Native peoples into the broader American society and to reduce federal obligations to tribes. In subsequent conversations with Elmer, he referred to Indigenous American communities as cultures of survival, explaining that despite federal policies and programs aimed at assimilation, Indigenous cultures continue to survive both in cities and on reservations. This theme of Native survival permeates Chicago's Indigenous community. While the Urban Indian Relocation Program's aim of assimilation was not met, it contributed to the growing migration of Native peoples from reservations to cities during the latter half of the twentieth century.

The Chicagoland area is currently home to tens of thousands of Indigenous Americans. An accurate estimate of the city's and the larger metropolitan area's Native population is a contested topic in the community. Community organizers argue that the United States Census Bureau grossly undercounts the city's Native population. Scholars have documented similar trends of undercounting of urban Native populations outside of Chicago in the late twentieth and early twenty-first centuries.[1] In 2019 the American Indian Center of Chicago estimated a population of sixty-five thousand Natives in the greater Chicago area, while the United States Census Bureau estimates just over fourteen thousand within the city limits.[2]

Chicagoland is the traditional homeland of the Meskwaki, Illinois, Kickapoo and Mascouten, Miami, Piankeshaw, Potawatomi, Sauk, Shawnee, and Winnebago peoples.[3] Like many geographical sites in the northern Midwest region of the United States, the roots of the city's name reach back to an Indigenous American term. Virgil Vogel traces the etymology of Chicago to the Miami Tribe's term for wild garlic, leek, or onion. Vogel additionally notes that the term Chicago is similar to the Illinois Tribe's term for "stinking beast," which may be why some believe the city name to mean "skunk place."[4] In 1832 and 1833 representatives of Indigenous American tribes in Illinois signed treaties ceding territory to the state of Illinois; the Native peoples of Illinois moved, and in some cases, were forcibly removed by military forces, to reservations outside the state, while the Chicago region was inhabited by white settlers.[5] The Chicago area remained Native territory to some degree; historian John N. Low documents the presence of the Pokagon Potawatomi in Chicago that has continued from the precontact era through the incorporation of Chicago as a city to the present day, demonstrating the important role the Potawatomi have played in the building of Chicago as a city.[6] In addition, the Native population of Chicago began to grow slowly in the early twentieth century, through urban migration, which increased in the 1930s, 1940s, and more significantly in the post–World War II era.

In this chapter I utilize interview data, archival material, and primary and secondary sources to meet four aims. First, I provide a brief history of the relationship between Indigenous American peoples and the United States federal government, beginning with the arrival of European settlers to the Americas. Second, I briefly discuss the migration of Indigenous Americans to Chicago in the early twentieth century. Third, I describe the efforts of United States politicians and legislators in the post–World War II era to reduce federal obligations to America's Indigenous nations and to assimilate Native peoples through a series of policies and programs. Fourth, I provide accounts from members of Chicago's Native community about what brought them to the city. Ultimately, my aim in this chapter is to introduce readers to the history of urban Indigenous American communities by looking at the motivations behind the migration of Native individuals and families to cities, while also documenting federal attempts to "get out of the Indian business" through the policies and programs of the 1950s. Throughout, the chapter begins to introduce readers to Chicago's Native community.

Shifting Policies from Assimilation to Sovereignty

A note before we begin—the experience of Indigenous American communities in relation to settler communities and the United States federal government is far from being a homogenous or simple one. What I describe is but a generalization of some of the larger historic events that do not completely describe the specific histories of any one group.

In the first several centuries after settler arrival in the New World—that is, the world "new" to those settlers—settler populations were dependent upon Indigenous Americans for survival and success in the unfamiliar landscape of North America. Settlers relied upon the Indigenous peoples for food and other resources, for knowledge of the North American landscape, and even for assistance in wars with opposing settler groups.[7] As Steven, a sixty-one-year-old Seneca man, explained in an interview:

> STEVEN: If it wasn't for them [the Native population of the region], the people that came to Virginia, they would have never made it because the Indians got them through that first winter, you know. And they had a big heart and stuff. We got all this land, you know, and they did, they gave them land and they fed them and stuff. And these Indians, they had a green thumb or something because they always had a bunch of corn and everything, and they were excellent hunters.

Steven explains that Indigenous people were adept at making a living in the North American landscape and that they assisted the newcomers in surviving in this new environment. As Steven's description reflects, though the Europeans were first dependent upon the Natives they encountered for survival, this relationship soon shifted.

By the time of the Revolutionary War, the American settler community had gained its footing in North America, while the diseases introduced into the Americas by settlers in concert with colonial policies were decimating the Indigenous population. Russell Thorn-

ton finds that smallpox, typhus, and measles were the most detrimental of the introduced diseases.[8] David Jones complicates the
simple "Virgin Soil" narrative proposed by Alfred Crosby, which
posits that Native populations were devastated by these diseases
due to the mere novelty of the conditions to the American conti-
nents and Indigenous bodies.[9] Jones instead shows that it was the
newness of these diseases coupled with the "turbulence of colonization" that led to the devastating outcomes for Native populations.[10] By 1789, several centuries after the arrival of European
settlers in the Americas, the settler community was less dependent
upon Indigenous Americans for survival; conversely, the latter were
devastated by disease and colonial encounters, and in some cases,
reliant upon settler resources.[11] For instance, Indigenous Americans turned to settler vaccines to combat the diseases brought from
Europe.[12] During the post–Revolutionary War era, the relationship
between the settler and Indigenous American communities began
to shift; in many instances it grew hostile as the new nation's desires
to spread further westward inevitably impinged on the life of local
communities. Since its founding, the United States has vacillated
between policies promoting the assimilation of Indigenous peoples and policies supporting Indigenous sovereignty.

In the United States, Indigenous tribal entities formed in relation to treaties and agreements with the federal government. Prior
to the arrival of European settlers, Indigenous American communities did not define themselves in terms of bounded tribal entities; rather, group membership was more fluid and based upon
a number of factors, including kinship and shared myth and ritual.[13] The term "tribe" referred traditionally to a group of people
who were politically autonomous and self-sufficient, who used
simple technology, who were not literate, and who had a distinct
culture, language, sense of identity, and religion. Anthropologist
Aiden Southall argued in 1970 that few groups meet this traditional definition of "tribe," and that in his experience working in
Africa, tribes were named in relation to other groups in the area
and shaped by the colonial state.[14] This holds true for Indigenous

American tribes. For example, the Tsistsistas are popularly recognized by the name Cheyenne, which is taken from the Sioux term meaning "red talkers," indicating for the Sioux a group of people who spoke a language they did not understand. Members of this community refer to themselves as Tsistsistas, which means "people" in their language.[15] It is true that contemporary Indigenous American nations use the terminology of "tribe," as do members of Chicago's Native community. Tribes today represent both ethnic and political groups; however, Indigenous American tribes are not representative of traditional conceptions of group identity; nor do they necessarily represent a cohesive group of peoples.[16]

While the relations between the federal government and Indigenous peoples of North America played a role in the development of tribal entities, the legal and political status of Indigenous American tribes has been and continues to be an ambiguous one in federal policies and laws. This ambiguous relationship began with the adoption of the United States Constitution in 1789. The commerce clause of the Constitution declares that "Congress shall have the power ... to regulate Commerce with foreign Nations, and among the several States, and with the Indian Tribes."[17] Tribes hold a unique position in the Constitution; while they stand as political entities alongside states and foreign nations, as indicated in their separate naming in the document, tribes are distinct from states and foreign nations. In Article VI, the Constitution defines tribes to be in a relationship with the federal government and not with state governments: "All treaties made, or which shall be made, under the authority of the United States shall be the supreme law of the land, and judges in every state shall be bound thereby."[18]

During the 1820s and 1830s a series of Supreme Court cases under Chief Justice John Marshall further delineated the United States–Indigenous American tribal relationship and the federal government's position on the sovereign status of tribes. The Marshall Trilogy defined tribes as wards of the United States federal government. Tribes were identified in these rulings as nations that were not permitted to sell their land to anyone but the federal government; they were also held to be outside the jurisdiction of state laws.[19] This ward-guardian relationship between the federal government and tribes is defined by a trust obligation, whereby the government has the duty to protect Indigenous American tribes. At the same time, this trust obligation obstructs complete tribal autonomy, and, moreover, the government does not always hold up its end of the deal.[20]

Since its founding, the federal government has neither solely focused on policies aimed at the assimilation of Indigenous American peoples nor defended and upheld Indigenous American sovereignty. President Andrew Jackson signed the Indian Removal Act in 1830 as well as seventy removal treaties during his term in office.[21] In some cases these treaties were not consented to by the larger majority of the tribal population, which led to events like the Trail of Tears of the Cherokee in 1838, the Trail of Death of the Potawatomi in the same year, and the 1864 Long Walk of the Navajo.[22] The reservation policy was not intended to go on indefinitely; the federal government expected Indigenous American peoples to assimilate over time into American society.[23]

To that end, the government put in place or supported a number of programs aimed at Indian assimilation during the nineteenth and early twentieth century. For example, the 1887 General Allotment Act, also known as the Dawes Act, divided up community shared reservation lands into family plots, which Indigenous Americans could sell after a period of time. The goal of allotment was to divide up Indigenous American peoples and break down their communities. It further reduced the amount of land Indigenous American tribes held collectively, returning excess land to the federal government, which in turn could sell it for a profit.[24] The tribal rolls that are a product of this allotment play an important role in tribal enrollment, which will be discussed in the next chapter.

A second program promoting assimilation, and which had devastating intergenerational effects on Native culture and life, involved boarding schools. The program stole Indigenous children from their families and transported them to the unfamiliar environment of an institutionalized boarding school. School administrators restricted children from using their Native language, taught them English, and encouraged them to assimilate into American society. These same administrators physically, emotionally, and sexually abused Indigenous children entrusted to their care.[25] This history of abuse and the corresponding low value placed on traditional Indigenous lifeways taught in this school system are histories that members of Chicago's Native community recall and reflect upon in interviews in this study.

The status of Indigenous American tribes as sovereign nations survived these attempts at assimilation and contributed to the continuing and growing tensions between Indigenous American tribes, state governments, and the federal government.[26] In the decades following World War I, the tide turned toward supporting Indigenous American sovereignty. The findings of the 1928 Meriam Report, which described the living conditions on reservations as deplorable, led to the passage of the 1934 Indian Reorganization Act, with the aim of Indian tribes becoming self-governing nations.[27] It was during this same era in the early twentieth century that some Indigenous Americans began migrating to urban areas.

Urban Migration in the Early Twentieth-Century Meriam Report

The Indigenous peoples of the Americas have built and inhabited urban centers for millennia, and Indigenous Americans have played important roles in the building of some contemporary cities in the United States, including Chicago and Seattle.[28] In the early decades of the twentieth century, a small number of Indigenous Americans migrated to urban spaces. The Meriam Report documented that the poor living conditions on reservations motivated individuals to migrate to urban areas in the first decades the century, and historians Rosalyn LaPier and David R. M. Beck explain that the boarding school system encouraged this trend.[29] Indigenous peoples who moved to urban areas in these years migrated for employment opportunities, and many of them found work in industry and service sectors, including agriculture, steel, railroads, resource extraction, and domestic labor.[30]

By the 1930s John Collier, at the time commissioner of the Office of Indian Affairs (OIA), sought to place Natives in wage-based employment near reservations to help benefit those communities through an influx of income.[31] The authors of the Meriam Report had described urban migration as an opportunity that could be mutually beneficial to reservation communities and urban centers, recommending that it be fostered as a policy of the OIA; Collier was implementing this proposed policy, in his case with the aim of finding employment for Natives near reservations to ensure income would return to improve the reservation economy.[32] An employee of the Office of Indian Affairs, Scott Henry Peters, a Chippewa businessman, worked with individuals to find employment in cities. He met with great success in placing Natives in jobs during the Depression while working out of the Chicago and Milwaukee offices from 1935–42.[33] Peters, however, was disciplined by the OIA because he found employment for individuals in urban spaces far from reservations instead of focusing on placing them in jobs locally, which ran counter to the prevailing policy.[34]

By the 1940s more and more Indigenous Americans were migrating to cities. In the context of the harsh poverty of reservation life, which had emerged out of over a century of policies and programs supported by the federal government, many Indigenous Americans opted to relocate to urban areas in search of stability and employment.[35] Deborah Davis Jackson's account of Native life in an unidentified midsize Midwestern city shows that many of those who moved there did so for the opportunity of employment in the booming automobile industry of the 1940s.[36] Historian Douglas K. Miller likewise demonstrates that many Natives moved to cities like Chicago both before and during the era of the Urban Indian Relocation Program for employment opportunities, particularly those in the war industry of World War II.[37]

In the years following the war, just over a decade after the Indian Reorganization Act was passed, the United States policies and programs were again focused on the assimilation of Indigenous Americans into the broader American society.

Postwar Era: Relocation and Aims of Assimilation

Beginning in the 1940s federal policies began to shift toward the promotion of Indigenous American assimilation with the aims of reducing the government's obligations to the tribes. According to geographer Tony Lazewski, the government was disappointed that the Indian Reorganization Act of 1934 did not provide more immediate results addressing the issues raised in the Meriam Report. In reaction to this disappointment, legislators developed policies and programs in the postwar era seeking to phase out the OIA.[38] The Urban Indian Relocation Program, which supported the migration of Indigenous Americans from reservations to cities, is one program among several during that era that were directed toward Indigenous American assimilation. Emerging in the late 1940s, both the Indian Claims Commission and the Zimmerman Plan aimed at ending federal obligations to Indigenous American tribes.[39] The Indian Claims Commission of 1946 was developed for tribes to bring past grievances to federal courts and to be compensated for past offenses against them. Geographer Elaine M. Neils explains that the underlying goal of the commission was for the government to end all claims on its services by adjudication through the courts.[40] Between 1946 and 1978, Indigenous American tribes won 58 percent of the cases brought to the commission; these tribes were awarded a total of $818 million through 546 claims cases.[41] The acceptance of federal reimbursement, however, threatened tribal sovereign status.[42]

In the year after the launch of the Indian Claims Commission, acting Indian Commissioner William Zimmerman sorted tribes into four categories, ordering them by what he thought was their level of preparedness for the withdrawal of federal services; this sorting became known as the Zimmerman Plan.[43] Historian Peter Iverson explains that Zimmerman's sorting was the result of his being put on the spot in a Senate committee hearing and being torn between the Senate's desire to scale back funding for the Bureau of Indian Affairs (as the OIA was known from 1949 onward) and his knowledge of the varied range of needs on reservations. The ramifications of Zimmerman's sorting, however, were great for the tribes he described as prepared for the reduction of federal services; these tribes, including for instance the Menominee and Klamath Nations, were among the first to lose these benefits.[44] Through termination policy the federal government abrogated its recognition of the affected Indigenous American nations' sovereign status. Donald Fixico refers to the Indian Claims Commission and the Zimmerman Plan as the germs of termination because these programs were precursors to the Termination and Urban Indian Relocation Programs of the 1950s—the Zimmerman Plan identified which tribes were prepared for assimilation and termination and the Indian Claims Commission threatened tribal sovereignty upon the acceptance of claims payments.[45]

In the early 1950s policies and congressional resolutions continued to support Indigenous American assimilation. In 1950 President Harry Truman appointed Dillon Myer to the position of commissioner of Indian Affairs. During the war, Myer had directed the relocation of Japanese Americans to internment camps. Kenneth Philp notes that Myer likened the quality of life on reservations at the time to that of a detention center.[46] As commissioner of Indian Affairs, Myer in 1952 launched efforts toward the development of the Urban Indian Relocation Program.[47] In 1953 the Eighty-Third Congress passed House Concurrent Resolution 108, laying the foundation for the termination of tribal sovereign status.[48] The resolution states: "It is declared to be the sense of Congress that, at the earliest possible time, all of the Indian tribes [listed on the resolution] and the individual members thereof . . . should be freed from federal supervision and control from all disabilities and limitations specifically applicable to Indians."[49] In framing the termination of tribal status as "freeing" individuals from supervision and control, the authors of this resolution gloss over the termination of tribal status in favor of highlighting the freedom it would bring individual tribe members.

Between 1945 and 1960, a total of 109 Indigenous American tribes were terminated across the United States under House Concurrent Resolution 108. This policy eliminated sovereign status and terminated the trust relationship between the federal government and the tribes.[50] (Since then, some of the terminated tribes have regained their former status, including both the Menominee and Klamath tribes.) On August 15, 1953, Public Law 280 was passed with no debate in Congress, effectively reducing federal involvement in Indigenous American tribal concerns.[51] This law turned criminal and civil jurisdiction of Indian tribes in six states and territories over to the state governments.[52] Even as power changed hands in Washington, the policies favoring Indigenous American assimilation in the postwar era did not shift. According to historian Larry Burt, Glenn Emmons, the commissioner of Indian Affairs under President Dwight Eisenhower, had developed an agenda for the gradual termination of all Indigenous American tribes by the bicentennial of the United States—July 4, 1976.[53] Generally speaking, the plans and actions of the commissioners of Indian Affairs and the laws and resolutions that passed through Congress in the decade following World War II show a general tendency favoring the termination of the trust obligation between the federal government and Indigenous American tribes; in place of this trust obligation, plans and programs oriented toward the assimilation of Indigenous American peoples were cultivated.

The Urban Indian Relocation Program, then, was one among several policies and programs during the postwar era that favored Indigenous American assimilation. As described above, in the decades before the development of the Urban Indian Relocation Program, Indigenous Americans migrated to cities in search of work.[54] During the war Indigenous Americans moved from reservations to cities both to work in factories supporting the war effort and to be in a central transportation hub if a family member in the service had leave time.[55] Assistance to reservations evaporated during the war years, further supporting migration.[56] During the war Natives enlisted in the United States military; of all eligible Indigenous men, 32 percent served in World War II as members of the armed forces.[57] Indigenous Americans have served and continue to serve in the United States Armed Forces in greater proportions than any other ethnicity in the United States.[58] Indigenous men and women voluntarily enlisted in the United States Armed Forces; according to participants in the Chicago American Indian Oral History Pilot Project, Indigenous Americans joined the World War II war effort as a means of following their people's tradition of warriors in a contemporary context.[59]

Based upon Dillon Myer's plans, the Bureau of Indian Affairs began to offer services to tribal members interested in relocating to urban areas in the early 1950s; the bureau initially offered financial assistance for housing and detailed employment officers who helped relocatees find work.[60] Nicolas G. Rosenthal describes that the idea for the Urban Indian Relocation Program originated in 1948, when the Bureau of Indian Affairs assisted Navajo and Hopi men to find work off the reservation after a rough winter limited their subsistence and work on reservation land.[61] Based upon these events, in 1950 the Navajo-Hopi Long Range Act was passed. This act not only supported the rehabilitation of Navajo and Hopi reservations through funding for education, health, construction, and resource development but also increased support for the relocation of Navajo and Hopi people to urban areas. In 1952 the bureau extended this program to other reservations.[62] That same year Congress appropriated $579,600 for the opening of field relocation offices in Los Angeles, Denver, and Chicago. This early start of the program offered relocating Indigenous Americans transportation to their urban destination, employment placement services in the city, financial assistance for subsistence needs before individuals received their first paycheck, and guidance in adjusting to city life.[63] The amount of money spent on each client who joined the Urban Indian Relocation Program increased over the several decades that the program was in place; according to Elaine M. Neils's research, the program on average spent $410 per client in 1955, $710 in 1960, $1,750 in 1965, and $2,270 in 1970.[64]

In order to relocate Indigenous Americans to cities, the Bureau of Indian Affairs set up field offices in large cities as well as near reservations around the country to encourage and recruit individuals to relocate.[65] In the early 1950s these agency offices collected materials documenting Native life on reservations; the data include typed notes on housing, education, religion, employment, and health status of individuals on reservations as well as photographic documentation of reservation life and struggles.[66] The Bureau of Indian Affairs agents who authored these documents strove to make relocation sound necessary while portraying the situation on the reservation as being without hope of recovery.

The agency offices' findings on the status of Native reservation life are summed up in the conclusion to the Great Lakes Agency's Brief History: "The conclusion which must be drawn then, is that many of the people do not have adequate opportunities on the reservations and the surrounding areas, and from this standpoint it is felt that the program of relocation services is indeed a boon to this needy group."[67] As a brief history explained earlier in the document, "The relocation division's basic objective is to facilitate the voluntary relocation of Indians who are unemployed or underemployed, to areas where there is steady employment and they have a chance to become self-supporting on a standard of living compatible with health and decency and to become part of the normal social and economic life of the nation."[68] In this vein, the agency offices across the Midwest and Northern Plains described the situation on reservations as bleak.

Despite the similarities between the 1928 Meriam Report and the Bureau of Indian Affairs field office reservation area reports, the responses differed greatly. While the Meriam Report led to the 1934 Indian Reorganization Act supporting Indian self-administration, the 1950s findings supported the Bureau of Indian Affairs' view that relocation was the best solution for the issues of poverty and unemployment faced by Indigenous Americans living on reservations. It is clear in the Great Lake Agency's documentation of its own history that the aims of relocation were to assimilate Indigenous Americans into American society, or what agency officials termed "normal social and economic life."[69] As the group wielding relative power, the officials of the Bureau of Indian Affairs and policymakers in Washington perceived their own way of life to be "normal," marking anything that did not mirror it as "abnormal" social life. The Urban Indian Relocation Program gained support from the agency offices' reports, which gave a figurative green light and provided moral justification for a program aimed at the assimilation of Native peoples into American society.

While the official line of the Bureau of Indian Affairs was that they supported the relocation of those who were most prepared to relocate, the reality was that the agency offices would send anyone willing to move to the city. An interviewee in the 1980s Chicago American Indian Oral History Pilot Project describes how he was asked one day if he would like to move to a city and found himself on a train to Chicago just a few days after this passing conversation with an agency officer.[70] Peter Iverson describes that among the Navajo who relocated in the 1950s, urban migrants included those least familiar with Anglo culture and language.[71]

Kurt Dreifuss, director of the Chicago Bureau of Indian Affairs office, explained the program to the *Chicago Daily Tribune* in a 1957 article reporting that "tribal families like suburban life:" "All who come here under the program make application before they leave the reservation and have assurances of jobs and housing. Upon arrival they are advised how to shop, health service is provided, and they receive a grant for initial purchases of food, housewares, and clothing."[72] Yet, though the Bureau of Indian Affairs promoted the Urban Indian Relocation Program as screening and preparing Natives to migrate to American cities, as noted above, anyone willing to relocate did so, without preparatory help.[73] Wade Arends's study of the program in the late 1950s demonstrates that its aim was purely assimilative. Those who relocated to Chicago were not notified of the existence of the American Indian Center of Chicago or other Native organizations and were scattered throughout the city to limit contact with other Indigenous people.[74]

Today, some members of Chicago's Native community reflect on the aims of the program with indignation. Elmer, quoted at the opening of this chapter, uses the strongest language of those I spoke with in reflecting upon the aims of relocation. From what he witnessed as a child during the early years of the program, Elmer characterizes the policy as a form of genocide, whose nefarious goals were achieved by moving Natives to cities where, in his view, the death of large numbers of Native peoples went unnoticed. Harriet, a second-generation Ojibwe relocatee, describes the program as an involuntary one that attempted to split up her family. Harriet, now fifty years old, retold the experience of her grandmother being forced into the program on the Lac du Flambeau Reservation:

> HARRIET: Well my mother, my grandmother who lived on a reservation in Wisconsin, she was brought here by the Relocation Act. And then her kids were put in foster homes on the reservation, until they all snuck away and they made their way here to Chicago to find their mother . . . She [her grandmother] was forced here. She was forced off the reservation.

Nicolas G. Rosenthal documents that pregnant women and single women with children were not typically accepted into the Urban Indian Relocation Program, and in the cases where single women with children did join the program, they were required to leave their children behind.[75] The program was unapologetically aimed at assimilating Native peoples into American society. Still, though Chicago Natives I spoke to were resoundingly angry about the underlying aims of assimilation, not everyone reflects on the program with the same anger as Harriet and Elmer. Many first-generation migrants describe the program as a boon to them and their families during that era, an aspect of this phenomenon that I examine more fully below.

The Urban Indian Relocation Program was largely successful in its aim of relocating a significant portion of the Native population from reservation areas to cities. Between 1952 and 1972 a hundred thousand Indigenous Americans relocated to urban cities from rural areas and reservations through the federally established program, and more people migrated without the assistance of the program to be near friends and family who had already migrated.[76] The Bureau of Indian Affairs assisted in the relocation of Indigenous Americans to Chicago, Cleveland, Dallas, Denver, Los Angeles, San Francisco, and San Jose during the early years of the plan and extended the locations to Tulsa and Oklahoma City by 1968.[77] According to 2010 census data, nearly 80 percent of Indigenous Americans live outside of reservation spaces, and the majority of those live in urban areas.[78] In the next section I look at what motivated people to move to Chicago.

Moving to the City

Frances and her late husband, both citizens of the Sisseton Wahpeton Sioux, moved from the Lake Traverse Reservation in South Dakota to Chicago in 1958. Now aged eighty-four after having raised her eleven children and worked for forty-five years in Chicago, Frances described why she and her husband chose to move through the Urban Indian Relocation Program:

> FRANCES: Oh we came on the relocation. They placed us here. We had a choice between Chicago and Los Angeles, but we took Chicago because you know it's closer to home, you can travel home and the other way would be too far and stuff, yeah . . . I thought it was good. Because that's the way you can learn to what trade they give you, schooling that you have to go take up, some kind of trade or something you know, that's one good thing. That's what my husband went under. He went, became a barber, he went to barber school. Yeah, they offer you jobs and stuff, school, training, training. That was good, I don't mind it. Otherwise we could have been living all the old ways yet. We came a long time ago when nothing was good over there [the reservation] yet, but now it is. Everything's all up to date like at home [the reservation].

Thus, in their decision to move to Chicago, Frances's family sought a locale that would be close to their home—which Frances continues to visit each year—in addition to providing opportunities for a better quality of life.

Indigenous Americans did not migrate merely because there were programs prepared to help them relocate; rather, those who came to cities did so for a variety of reasons. In this section I utilize oral history interview data in concert with archival material and secondary sources to show that individuals who chose to move and to stay in cities considered multiple and overlapping factors in making their decisions. While the Urban Indian Relocation Program assisted some in their migration to Chicago, many more Indigenous Americans moved to the city on their own. Of the twenty-nine oral history interview participants in this study, three moved to Chicago through the Urban Indian Relocation Program, eighteen moved to Chicago on their own, and eight were born in the city. Of those born in Chicago, seven knew the history of their family's migration to the city; five were born in the city because their parents or grandparents moved to Chicago through the program and two because their parents moved there on their own. The majority of participants in the 1980s Chicago American Indian Oral History Pilot Project described choosing to move to Chicago in search of better opportunities.[79] In speaking of what led them to move to Chicago, they described how the opportunities on the reservations were scarce while the city had ample job prospects. Participant responses here mirror those of the Pilot Project—in both cases, opportunities in the city appeared to far exceed those on the reservation and drew many individuals and families to relocate.

Forty-six thousand Indigenous Americans left reservations for wartime work in cities during World War II.[80] The Urban Indian Relocation Program only increased the rate of Indigenous American relocation. Though this program was supposed to be voluntary, in that no one was forced against their will to relocate, it was also involuntary in the sense that economic help on reservations was greatly scaled back during this period; the federal government was offering multiple services in the designated relocation cities while reducing programming on reservations.[81] The Bureau of Indian Affairs agents at reservation field offices presented to reservation Natives images of city life that appeared desirable in contrast to the one they knew. Posters, informational handouts, and advertisements portrayed cities as welcoming Indigenous Americans and offering opportunities for training, employment, housing, family life, and financial security. Scholars have documented the misleading nature of these advertisements.[82] Participants in Wade Arends's study, for instance, described that a family photographed as an example of "successful relocation" had moved in fact back to the reservation. A participant in his interviews describes being dressed up as a butcher for a photoshoot for one such advertisement to be used on his home reservation, because his friends back home knew that he had hoped to find work as a butcher in the city.[83]

As Frances described in her statement above, there were fewer employment opportunities on her reservation in South Dakota in the late 1950s than there are today, and the same was true for many reservations across the United States at that time. Alan Sorkin describes the economic situation of reservations in the mid-1960s as one of abject poverty, explaining that the median income on all reservations was below and the unemployment rates were above the median income and unemployment rates of the rest of the nation.[84] This economic situation promoted the migration of many Natives to urban spaces. Almeda is a seventy-seven-year-old Choctaw woman who moved to Chicago in 1961, having followed her then-boyfriend and future husband to the city. Almeda described the hardship she faced on the Mississippi Choctaw Reservation near Philadelphia, Mississippi, even though, like the Lake Traverse Reservation described by Frances, the situation on her reservation has greatly improved in recent years:

ALMEDA: I think it [the Urban Indian Relocation Program] did a lot of good for a lot of people, because it was, you know Philadelphia, Mississippi, is such a small town, and [there were] not that many jobs at that time.

The job scarcity and low employment rates Frances and Almeda saw on their reservations during the 1950s and 1960s were two of many issues faced by Natives living on reservations; other problems included poor housing conditions, low quality food, limited access to higher quality foods and medical care, and high rates of alcoholism. As I will describe in chapter 3, the commodity food supplies provided by the United States government have played a significant role in the growing rates of diabetes and obesity among Native peoples today.[85] While the economic situation on many reservations has improved since the mid-twentieth century, for much of the second half of the twentieth century the living conditions on the reservations were poor. During this period Indigenous Americans moving to cities were actively engaged in life choices aimed at survival.

There were other difficulties beyond unemployment on reservations that prompted individuals to relocate to cities. Two interviewees in this study spoke of distancing themselves from physically and emotionally abusive family relations on the reservation. The decision to move to escape abuse was also reported by participants in the 1980s Oral History Pilot Project.[86] High rates of alcoholism were another aspect of reservation life that some families hoped to leave behind in migrating to a city. Sandra, a sixty-one-year-old San Carlos Apache woman, described how her father participated in the Urban Indian Relocation Program in 1954 as a means of moving his family away from what she described as a dangerous environment for her mother, who was then battling alcoholism:

> SANDRA: My father came out of the service and then he wanted to move to the c[ity], get away from the reservation because it was too many drinking going on. He tried to get my mother away from there so we moved to Phoenix, but it didn't work, so he took a part in the Relocation Act and they asked him what city would he like to go to, and he had his choice of cities that he can go to. So he chose Chicago, and then we all came on a train over here. And the Bureau of Indian Affairs helped us get situated by finding my dad a job and food, furniture, clothing, and whatever necessities we needed, they helped. And then we were here, my father and my family had to be on our own after that.

Unfortunately for Sandra's family, moving to Chicago did not resolve her mother's addiction to alcohol.[87] Sandra described how she dropped out of high school to take on the role of homemaker, raising her younger siblings and cooking for her family while her dad worked the third shift and her mother continued to struggle with her condition. Alcohol addiction has been and continues to be a significant social and health concern in urban Native communities.[88] In Chicago, oral history interview participants describe how there were "bars galore" in neighborhoods where Natives lived and that some establishments in those areas came to be known as "Indian bars." Bars were a space for socialization in those early decades. Building on this point, one interviewee in this study added that Indigenous Americans also socialized at the all-Native churches that sprang up in cities across the United States during this period.

While the twenty-nine oral history interviewees had multiple reasons for moving to Chicago, finding employment was a primary factor for eighteen of them. In contrast to employment opportunities on reservations, jobs in Chicago during the era of the Urban Indian Relocation Program were abundant, and people did not have to move through the program itself to find work in cities like Chicago. Agnes, an eighty-two-year-old Odawa woman, moved to Chicago for work in 1958. Though Agnes worked at only two places during her forty-one years of working life there, she described how easy it was to find work when she first moved to the city:

AGNES: I just wanted to move on. So I came here. Oh jobs were so plentiful . . . You could work at one job and if you didn't like it, walk out and you'd have another one tomorrow. But I stayed with mine.

The oral history interview participants worked a variety of jobs with widely different training and educational requirements. Those I spoke with worked as factory workers, truck drivers, daily pay employees, office workers, pharmacy technicians, nurses, employment officers, police dispatchers, customer service representatives, and employees of Native organizations in the city, including the

American Indian Center of Chicago and the Anawim Center (now known as the Saint Kateri Center of Chicago).

The high demand for workers that Agnes describes continued for those who migrated to Chicago throughout the early 1980s. In describing how she and her husband moved to Chicago in 1979, Susan, a fifty-eight-year-old Seneca woman, explained how they had intended to move to Texas, where her husband, Steven, could find work as a welder on an oil rig:

> SUSAN: Actually we were on our way to Texas. We were going to go because they needed welders down there and that's what he did. I was working at Fisher Price in New York when we left. I quit my job and packed up and we were on our way there but then we had a . . . one of his cousins lived here and she's like, well just stay for the weekend and then this, the construction job came up for him and they hired him like the next Tuesday, so, and we've been here ever since.

The abundance of jobs in Chicago from World War II to the early 1980s stood in stark contrast to the lack of job opportunities and generally poor living conditions found on many reservations during the same period, drawing many Natives to the Windy City. According to local employment officers from the Chicago branch of California Manpower Consortium, however, Natives currently face high rates of unemployment in the city, while on some, though not all, reservations opportunities for employment are increasing.

In addition to jobs and a desire for a better life, other factors contributed to people's motivations, including interest in nearness to family, Indigenous American activism, and chance opportunity. Consideration of distance from family and home reservations was an important factor for those who migrated to Chicago. While some intentionally moved far away from family, as noted above in cases of abuse, others like Susan and Almeda first came to Chicago to see or to be near family. Sylvia, a sixty-nine-year-old woman who was born on the Leech Lake Chippewa Reservation in Minnesota, described how she and her entire family slowly migrated to Chicago:

> SYLVIA: My sister was living here and, and one by one we were leaving for the city and my sister finally came and she said come on home with me, come back to Chicago with me, and I said well I, I said that's too big of a city. (laughs) . . . She said come on! She coaxed me, so I said okay I'll go with you. Then my [other] sister came, then my brother, my sister and brother were already here. So well most of us were here by then. Then my mother came last.

Sylvia lived in Chicago until her death several years ago with, as she put it, more grandchildren than she could count, after first arriving in the city in 1959. For many relocatees, being near the home reservation and family also factored into the city choice in relocating—as seen in Frances's description of how she and her husband chose Chicago over Los Angeles. Many first-generation relocatees visit their home reservation one or more times a year to see family, seek medical care, and participate in their nation's cultural and political activities. They pass this practice of visiting on to younger generations, who first join their parents on visits in childhood and then begin to visit the reservation on their own and with their families as they grow older.

Employment and proximity to family and home reservation were important factors for those who migrated to cities, but the initial move could be sparked by a wide variety of individual interests and experiences. In the 1970s Randall was drawn to Chicago after having read about his cousin's involvement in the Chicago Indian Village—an act of protest against the poor housing conditions many Native people of Chicago faced at that time.[89] Now sixty-eight, Randall was almost thirty years old when he moved to Chicago from the Menominee Reservation in 1974:

> RANDALL: I saw on the news, I think it was in the paper, a cousin of mine was demonstrating outside of Wrigley Field, and I wanted to come down here to see what was going on.

While Randall did not actively take part in the Chicago Indian Village protests, he did continue to live in the city after finding work. In a 2010 conversation another interviewee, named Tammy, mentioned that she had moved to Chicago on a dare. Tammy is a sixty-eight-year-old woman who moved from the Oneida reservation outside of Green Bay, Wisconsin, to Chicago in 1961. She elaborated upon this event in an interview we completed in December 2012:

> TAMMY: I was twenty-one when I first came here and what brought it down here [was a] bunch of us kids out joyriding. They went back the next day. I was only one out of six of them that stayed—from Green Bay . . . I stayed and the other ones went home.

Similar to other interviewees, Tammy had no trouble finding work once she arrived in Chicago and she chose to stay in the city until she passed away in 2013.

Not everyone who relocated chose to remain in the city. Alfred is an eighty-seven-year-old Turtle Mountain Chippewa man who was born in North Dakota. Alfred moved to Chicago on his own in 1953 after hearing from his brother in the city about the work there. Alfred's future wife and brother moved to Chicago through the Urban Indian Relocation Program, and he described the program as beneficial for many Indigenous Americans who moved through its assistance. While Alfred lived in Chicago for sixty years before our interview, he described how another of his brothers did not adjust to city life and returned to their reservation in North Dakota:

> ALFRED: A lot of Indians went back, a lot of them . . . My brother from Belcourt, they sent him to California. And that's what they promised him. He had four kids. Finding those jobs, find you a job, you get a check, you pay for your bills, but [after] the first paycheck, you're on your own. So he stayed there one year . . . [He said] I get my check, I pay the rent, I pay for this, [and] there's nothing to even feed my family. He said to hell with that, so he came home.

Alfred's brother's experience in California was not unlike that of many others. According to correspondence sent by Gerard Littman to Father Peter Powell—a priest at St. Augustine's Center for the American Indian who dedicated his life to running this religious organization from the mid-1950s to the late 2010s—in the early 1960s there were nine thousand Indigenous Americans settled in Chicago. At the same time, there were between fourteen thousand and sixteen thousand in the city at some point during the year, with as many as 40 percent returning home after attempting city life for a year or less.[90]

Natives faced other challenges besides the purely financial after relocating to cities. The most significant was that of loneliness in the city space. While loneliness prompted many relocatees to return to the reservation, it also led to the development of Native community centers.[91] As already mentioned, participants in this study describe that other sites for socializing included both bars and churches. Another challenge involved bias in job placement and job training. The Bureau of Indian Affairs sponsored training for blue-collar work, but not for college education or white-collar employment.[92] While the Urban Indian Relocation Program was aimed at the assimilation of Indigenous Americans into American society, the bureau did not strive to assimilate Indigenous Americans into middle-class white American society.

Finding clean affordable housing was a further challenge. The Bureau of Indian Affairs' aim was to scatter Indigenous Americans around urban areas, but the housing situation in cities thwarted this goal.[93] On the West Coast, for example, the government office had planned to disperse Indigenous Americans around the San Francisco Bay Area by housing them in apartments far from one another; the agency had hoped thereby to prevent tribal contact and promote assimilation. However, due to limited budgets, the bureau could barely afford to house Indigenous Americans in apartments, let alone separate apartment buildings around the Bay. In the end, the Bureau of Indian Affairs created all-Indian apartment complexes, thereby failing to meet their original intent.[94] In the case of Chicago, by the 1970s, Uptown—a northeast community area bordering Lake Michigan—was known throughout the city as the "Indian neighborhood."[95] According to James LaGrand, by the late 1950s "Uptown [had] achieved a special status in the minds of Indians in Chicago. It was the place to be with other Indians."[96] Those who relocated faced problems with the houses and apartments themselves, ranging from unclean homes with broken windows, mold, and roach infestations to homes that were too small to fit large families.[97] This experience was not an uncommon one; rather, many found that through participating in the Urban Indian Relocation Program, they had traded rural poverty for urban slums.[98] This poor housing situation prompted a group of Indigenous Americans to protest against living conditions in Chicago's northside Wrigleyville neighborhood in the 1970s.[99] Housing discrimination is still a concern today. In the early 2000s a landlord in the northwest side of the city told interviewee Tammy that by policy he does not rent his properties out to Native Americans, not recognizing when he spoke to her that she was herself of Native descent.

Though Alfred's brother chose to move back home upon finding it nearly impossible to maintain his family on his city income, many others who migrated from the reservation to the city and back to the reservation did so multiple times. Joshua first moved to Chicago in his thirties for work, but he was no stranger to living in an urban area. Joshua, sixty-four at the time of our interview, moved with his family in and out of the White Earth Chippewa Reservation in Minnesota many times in his childhood:

> JOSHUA: I grew up many places. I grew up on the White Earth Reservation till I was about seven or eight and then we moved through Indian Relocation Act, which is a government policy to, to assimilate Native Americans and moved to urban Indian areas where the Bureau of Indian Affairs would place my father into a job and get us an apartment and then after a couple months, we'd be on our own. So we moved to Minneapolis, things didn't work out. We went back to the reservation. Then we moved to Los Angeles. Things didn't work out there, so we came from California back to Billings, Montana, where my other uncle had obtained a job

in construction and offered to see if he could get my dad a job in construction, and he, they did. So we lived in Billings, Montana, for a year after Los Angeles, and then we moved from there back to Minnesota and then we moved to Milwaukee. And then I went through high school and college in Milwaukee.

Experiences like Joshua's were not uncommon. Orlando Garcia describes that many who migrated to the Chicago area during the era of the Urban Indian Relocation Program moved multiple times.[100] While some scholars describe this trend to be a result of the failure of the Bureau of Indian Affairs to adequately prepare people to move to the city, it may be more complicated than these explanations assume.[101] Instead of considering this as a failing system of relocation, it might also be looked at as Native peoples seeking out the opportunities that best met their own desires and needs—whether to be nearer to family, to be nearer to their reservation, to be able to find work, to gain an education in a specific field, or to be closer to a vibrant and active intertribal Native community.

As already mentioned, while a great number of Native people migrated with the assistance provided by the Urban Indian Relocation Program, many others made their way to the city on their own. Reasons for the move ranged from wanting to get away from problems on the reservation, greater employment opportunities in cities, the desire to be near family members who were already in cities, and supporting Indigenous American activism. While second-generation relocatee Harriet describes her family's relocation as one of forced movement, nearly all first-generation relocatees describe a more agentive role in moving to the city to survive and find work. This survival, of course, was survival from the detrimental policies that led to extreme unemployment and harsh living conditions on reservations. The choice to remain in the city was and continues to be influenced by employment opportunities, family relationships, and opportunities to participate in urban Indigenous American activities, which have promoted and enabled the long-term residence of many Chicago Natives.

The greater Chicagoland area is home today to a large Indigenous American population. According to the American Indian Center, this population includes individuals representing more than one hundred tribes. The participants in this study represent a small sample of this population. These participants self-identify as citizens from twenty-six tribes across the United States and Canada, including Apache, Akimel O'odham, Arikara, Assiniboine, Cherokee, Chippewa, Choctaw, Covelo, Dakota, Ho-Chunk, Lakota, Menominee, Meskwaki, Micmac, Navajo, Odawa, Ojibwe, Omaha, Oneida, Ponca, Potawatomi, Pueblo, Sac and Fox, Seneca, Sioux, and Stockbridge. Participants agree that the Native population of Chicago has decreased over the last few decades, citing that some are moving further into the suburbs, some are dying, and others are moving back to reservations. Uptown is no longer the "Indian neighborhood" it once was in the 1970s. Today Natives live throughout the city and its surrounding areas. The American Indian Center has found through census and demographic research that a significant majority of the city's Natives live in the Irving Park and Portage Park neighborhoods, just a few miles west of Uptown. In 2017 the center relocated from its building on Wilson Avenue in Uptown to a new location on Ainslie Street in the Albany Park neighborhood, a few blocks north of Irving Park, to be nearer the residences of the majority of the Chicago Indigenous population. Though many first- and second-generation relocatees in this study continue to refer to the reservation as home, some Chicago Natives describe the city as their home. Steven, a sixty-one-year-old Seneca man who moved to Chicago in 1979, described his bond with the city based upon his time and construction career in the city:

> STEVEN: To me, it's my life, you know. Like I told you, I built this city, you know what I mean. To me it's got, means more than just being in the city. I can look at something and I know how that thing started and I know how it was built and or even like I said I can take the grandchildren and show them the Shedd Aquarium and we reconstructed Lake Shore drive . . . I had the chance to do

stuff like this and this is stuff that I'll remember forever, and even, even I've passed it onto my grandchildren. My grandchildren are proud to say hey my grandfather did you know this and this and built this and that you know what I mean. It's, that's why I love this city so much you know, cause to me it's like in my blood, you know.

The programs and policies of the United States federal government from the nineteenth century to the postwar era played a role in motivating the migration of Indigenous Americans from across the United States and Canada to Chicago. The urban experience that Indigenous Americans faced upon arrival through the Bureau of Indian Affairs' Urban Indian Relocation Program proved to be a harsh and alienating encounter with the society into which the government hoped Indigenous Americans would assimilate. In reality Indigenous Americans who relocated to cities did not passively assimilate into American city life, as policy makers in Washington DC had hoped; they participated in intertribal alliances and activities and maintained tribal contacts, effectively reasserting Native identity in an urban context while making a home in the city. In the next chapter I utilize interview materials, along with findings from archival research and secondary sources, to discuss contemporary Indigenous American identity and community in Chicago.

2

Native Chicago

C hatting on the turquoise velvet couch in the Little One's room of the American Indian Center, I asked Rosanna, a twenty-eight-year-old Oneida woman, what it means to be Native in a city like Chicago. A few weeks earlier, the Lakota Grandmother Truth Tour, a group of documentary filmmakers and Lakota citizens from the Pine Ridge Reservation, had come to the center to screen the poignant documentary *Red Cry*. The film documents the history of colonialism and the detrimental effects it continues to have on the Lakota of Pine Ridge. More than forty Chicago Natives attended the screening and discussion that Friday night. The atmosphere shifted over the course of the evening, moving from excitement for the event, to grief upon hearing about the past and current situation on Pine Ridge, and finally to anger and unease when the reservation Natives in the film and in the conversation that followed described urban Natives as having lost their culture in the city space. Within five days of the film screening, the center held a healing circle—a gathering in which community members shared their feelings about the event with the aim of resolving and coming to terms with the issues it brought up. In the interim, conversations in person and on social media arose in which Chicago Natives voiced their anger over the way in which the film and the

Truth Tour representatives spoke of urban Natives. In response to my question on Native identity in the city, Rosanna voiced her disagreement with the views expressed by the visitors to the center that April evening:

> ROSANNA: Other people might think we're assimilated, we don't know our culture, we don't know about being Native, but since, I mean, I don't think that's ever been true. I think people struggle with that a lot, but I think no matter what, we still have different worldviews and ways of relating to the world no matter where we are . . . Our original medicines still come through the cracks of pavements, so like we, our animal and plant relatives are here with us, like we're not devoid of that. It's always been here.

Urban Natives stand in a unique position. They are, as Rosanna describes, enmeshed in city life while also embodying and enacting Native identity in an urban space. Rosanna's response challenges the notion that urban Natives have assimilated, as the designers of the Urban Indian Relocation Program had intended or as some reservation Natives believe they have. In reality, urban Natives enact and cultivate their culture and traditions in individual households and as part of larger tribal and intertribal networks.

Chicago's contemporary Indigenous population is diverse; it is multigenerational and multitribal, made up of individuals whose ancestors originated in distant geographic locations; moreover, it consists of a diverse range of economic standings. As noted in the previous chapter, participants in this study self-identified as citizens of twenty-six tribes. In turn, they are one small sample of the greater Chicagoland Native population, which is estimated to represent more than one hundred tribes from across the United States and Canada. In this chapter I describe Chicago's Native community. First, I explore concepts and enactments of Native identity in the city space. As reflected in the description of the film screening at the American Indian Center, there is significant pressure on the urban population to identify as Native. This pressure comes not only from those living on reservations but also from both Natives and non-Natives in the city space. Engaging with anthropological and sociological scholarship, I demonstrate that history, politics, and interactions with non-Natives inform and contribute to concepts of Native identity in Chicago. Finally, I describe Chicago's Native community, illustrating that it is made up of several interconnected networks that reach beyond the city to reservation spaces. While the community pulls together in times of need, there are also periods of division and infighting.

Politics, History, and Blood

The space in the conference room at Barry's place of work was cool and dimly lit. We sat at one end of a large conference table, on wheeled black pleather chairs that appeared and felt as though they were fresh from a warehouse. An hour into our interview, Barry abruptly left the room, returning moments later with two tribal identification cards from his office; as he showed them to me, he stated that he was proud to be a "card-carrying Indian." Barry, a sixty-eight-year-old Choctaw man who has lived in several cities around the United States, contrasted his pride in having his tribal identification cards at hand with the attitudes of people he describes as scornfully claiming "I'm not a card-carrying Indian." Barry and I had deviated from our interview on diabetes and had been talking about the Affordable Care Act and the effect it would have on programs like the Indian Health Service, which led us into a discussion of how American Indian Health Service of Chicago (AIHSC) requires that people bring in a tribal identification card to demonstrate eligibility for services. As Barry explained, he was able to prove his ancestry and obtain a card, whereas those people he referred to in negative terms have not done the work to show that they are Native.

I had learned in the summer of 2012, a year before this interview with Barry, the importance people place on obtaining tribal identification cards in Chicago's Native community. Early that summer Rebecca gave special attention to instructing me on where to direct people with questions on how to trace Indigenous heritage while training me to respond to phone calls and emails while I volunteered at the American Indian Center's reception desk. The center, I soon learned, is contacted several times a week by individuals around the city who are trying to either trace their ancestry or to gather documentation to enroll as a citizen of a tribe. Rebecca explained that the person will first need to have some idea of what nation they descend from, and then learn the process of locating ancestry for that tribe. In most cases, she explained, citizenship can be proven by locating an ancestor on a roll, like the Dawes Roll. Rolls listing tribal citizens were created in the decades around the turn of the twentieth century, dating initially to the General Allotment Act of 1887. The method Rebecca described reflects the requirements of only some tribes, including the Cherokee, a tribe the center receives many inquiries about. For this reason, Rebecca explained that the center directs individuals with questions regarding ancestry either to the specific tribe directly or to the Newberry Library, which houses copies of some of these documents in the city and can better assist the callers. Chicago Natives who know their ancestry and whose children meet tribal requirements enroll their children in their tribes often within a short period after birth, a practice that has been in place in Chicago for several decades.[1]

Federally recognized tribes determine their own rules for citizenship, which vary by tribe. As historian Melissa Meyer explains, in setting the standard for enrollment, selection of the "variables that are ultimately employed is an arbitrary decision, but the implications for American Indians can be enormous."[2] Most tribes require ¼ blood quantum, meaning that, for instance, an individual must have one grandparent who is a full-blood tribal member to enroll as a citizen in the tribe.[3] Eva Garroutte and Kim Tallbear explain that while the European concepts of race and blood were first introduced within just the past few centuries, they permeate discussions of Native citizenship.[4] Prior to contact with Europeans, Indigenous Americans had their own systems for categorizing and marking the differences between groups of people.[5] In terms of blood and tribal citizenship, Kim Tallbear notes that while the federal government does not require federally recognized tribes to use blood quantum as a factor in the enrollment of citizens, the Bureau of Indian Affairs offers information to tribes on how to determine this factor, further propagating this form of identification.[6]

As Rebecca explained to me in 2012, the process of proving blood quantum often rests upon locating ancestors on a list like the Dawes Roll. Historian Alexandra Harmon demonstrates that studies on Indigenous American citizenship policies would greatly benefit from investigation of how tribes and federal agents determined who could and could not be included in a tribe's roll a century or more ago. In her study of the Coleville Roll, Harmon shows a discursive back and forth between federal agents' definitions of tribal membership and Indigenous definitions, in which federal agents focused on descent-based membership whereas tribal members considered kinship, residence, and behavior as important factors for inclusion.[7]

Blood, then, in this context is complicated and, to echo Harmon's call, more studies on the processes involved in the creation of rolls would be incredibly beneficial to understanding this aspect of tribal citizenship in the present. As anthropologist and science and technology studies scholar Kim Tallbear describes, though blood and forms of genetic evidence are shaped by and deeply enmeshed in social and political histories, the history of their making has been fetishized and many tribes and individuals incorporate these concepts of blood—and more recently—genetic evidence into their definitions of identity and citizenship.[8] While blood is recognized by Harmon and Tallbear to be a dubious marker of identity due to this social and political history, it is not often challenged or questioned within Native communities like that of Chicago. In Chicago, blood is referenced in discussions of Native identity, while genes are not. Blood is considered a substance through which identity is passed directly, a relationship I discuss in detail below.

While Indigenous American nations determine who can and cannot enroll as tribal citizens, the federal government wields significant power in determining which groups it recognizes as tribes.

Professor of social work Hilary Weaver explains that Native identity is defined in three ways—by the self, by the community, and by external identification. This external identification, she continues, is a form of power and exclusion.[9] Today the government plays a primary role in defining which groups are federally recognized as tribes and which are not. Historian James Clifford elaborates on this in his discussion of the 1977 *Mashpee Tribe v. New Seabury et al.* case and builds upon discussions of the meaning indigeneity in contemporary times. In this trial, the Mashpee sought recognition of their ownership of land based on the 1790 Non-Intercourse Act, which required congressional approval for any transfer of land from Indigenous to non-Indigenous holders. As Clifford demonstrates, the trial was more about the negotiation of Mashpee indigeneity than about the land dispute with the Seabury Company, which was reaping a substantial profit from its development of Cape Cod. In describing the efforts of the Mashpee, who lost this battle and their first appeal, Clifford explains that the court played the role of philosopher, defining who Natives are by interrogating contemporary Mashpee performances of indigeneity by the yardstick of the past.[10]

The power of the federal government in this context is a clear example of identity politics. Jonathan Hill and Thomas Wilson theorize the relationship between politics and identity as follows: "'Identity politics' refers mainly to the 'top down' processes whereby various political, economic, and other social entities attempt to mold collective identities, based on ethnicity, race, language and place, into relatively fixed and 'naturalized' frames for understanding political action and the body politic. 'Politics of identity' refers to a more 'bottom up' process through which local people challenge, subvert, or negotiate culture and identity and contest structures of power and wealth that constrain their social lives."[11] While both identity politics and politics of identity are at play in definitions of Native identity in Chicago, the politics of identity on the ground are fraught with more disagreement than Hill and Wilson's definition implies.

Whether one is Native or not can be challenged by other members of the community. After one senior lunch at the center, a newcomer spoke with several regulars about Native items he had an interest in selling. One elder who overheard this conversation walked past the newcomer muttering under her breath in a not-so-subtle way "You're no Indian." Locally, politics of identity are full of internal challenges, wherein pressure from inside the community is present and not just to do with tribal enrollment.

In addition to tribal enrollment, blood and appearance are important factors in some definitions of Native identity, even though blood in this context has a complicated social and political history. Lisa Oritz's early twenty-first-century survey of Chicago Natives' perception of identity found that for both "full-" and "mixed-blooded" Natives, blood and appearance are considered significant factors in determining whether or not one is Native.[12] I found that these two factors continue to be important today. Several people described a sense of pride in their status as full-blood members of a single tribe, while others expressed concern for the future due to genetic admixture of Native and non-Native peoples. Pauline, a fifty-seven-year-old Lakota woman, has lived her entire life in cities; she explained that it was important for both her and her mother to marry within the Native community and expressed concern over younger generations who are not doing the same. For Pauline, the Urban Indian Relocation Program's aims of assimilation were in a sense met by moving Natives to cities, where they would begin to partner with non-Natives:

PAULINE: Well I think they did their job. Their job was to break us up and to get us assimilated into you know a different culture and to probably make us extinct, and I think you know they're on their way. We, see like me and my sisters and my brother, we all have Indian kids, but their kids are half, so it's like, you know.

Earlier in our conversation, Pauline noted that she sees Native physical features fading away in the younger generations of her own family:

PAULINE: I kind of had that mindset too that I was going to marry a Native and nobody else, so he's Menominee. So he's Menominee, so my kids are Indian. You know, you know, so okay, so they're not half or whatever, so but my daughter, my middle one, her husband is white, I mean, so my granddaughter who's my granddaughter, you wouldn't even know she was mine. But no, she has blonde hair and the bluest eyes you've ever seen. Right, and then the other one, she looks like you [fair skin, dark hair, green eyes], so, so you know she's darker than the other one is, but the other one's blonde-haired and I mean the most beautiful blue eyes you've ever seen. And the other one has your color eyes and your color hair, maybe a little lighter, and they used to think that my daughter was their nanny. Nanny? That's her kids, her biological kids. But so then I got this one here is my youngest one and you can tell, she's African American, so you know I can't say anything because my kids, I do not have, I don't consider, I don't have any Native American–looking grandkids.

For Pauline, relationships producing children with less Native blood and phenotypic features are a physical marker of assimilation. Circe Sturm describes that views like Pauline's are shared on reservations; for example, on the Cherokee Reservation genetic mixing is seen as contributing to cultural loss.[13]

In Chicago, Natives marry fellow citizens of their own tribe, citizens of other Native nations, and non-Natives. There are challenges that come from marrying outside one's tribe; for instance, it is more difficult to enroll a child born in intertribal partnerships. In an article in Northwestern University's *Medill Reports*, Chicago Native community member Jasmine Gurneau describes some drawbacks to current processes of enrollment. She explains that her children do not meet the blood quantum requirements to be enrolled in either her or her spouse's tribes: "They are Oneida, Menominee and Ojibwe . . . even though they are not officially recognized by the tribes as citizens."[14] At the same time, marriages outside one's group can be beneficial in other ways, for instance in the promotion of intertribal understanding. While blood and physical inheritance are important factors in definitions of Native identity in Chicago today, definitions of Native identity both in the city and on reservations are fluid and incorporate many factors beyond blood and appearance.[15] Additional considerations in Native Chicago include kinship, spiritual practices, knowledge of and ability to speak Native languages, behavior, and shared history, values, and symbols.

Identity as Shared History and Experience

Group membership can be defined by the sharing of features— for instance, sharing a language, a cosmology, a set of ancestors, or an experience. The history of oppression throughout the past several centuries represents a set of shared experiences binding Native Chicagoans together. While today parents teach their children about Native culture and history, in the past this teaching was not always done openly or in many cases at all. Community members attribute this history of not passing on traditions to the experiences their parents and grandparents faced in boarding schools, where children were punished for speaking their Native languages and practicing their traditions. Larry, a fifty-three-year-old member of the Covelo Tribe, explained how the situation has shifted in recent years:

> LARRY: When I grew up because of the, the Indian school structure, the elders back then and my parents did not want their kids to be raised Native because they all had horrible experiences with it. So my generation had to find kind of its own way, and we had to reinvent. So it's nice to see some of the elders that are still around finally realizing I can't die without passing on my knowledge. So there's been a big explosion here I think in culture that I haven't seen before. And there's been some political strengthening of the group.

As Larry describes, a history of oppression led to a fear for survival. Several elders spoke of not teaching or learning Native culture or tradition either in the city or on the reservation.

Alfred, an eighty-seven-year-old member of the Turtle Mountain Chippewa, told me that he and his wife did not raise their children in their Native ways or engage them with other Natives in the Chicago area:

ALFRED: My kids they're here. I didn't raise mine Indian. I didn't raise my kids with Indian people until lately . . . They don't understand Indian. They don't speak my language, all English. That's terrible. Nobody thought to. Raise them like white kids.

Now later in life, Alfred expresses regret for not having taught his children his language and postponing involvement with the intertribal community of Chicago.

This practice of not teaching Native traditions to children was also found on some reservations during the mid-to-late twentieth century. Randall, a sixty-eight-year-old Menominee man, explained that the younger generations did not participate in ceremonies and traditional practices on his reservation, and consequently he could not learn pieces of his culture until later in life:

RANDALL: Well as a younger child when I was growing up, I would go, our parents would take us to reservation where they had powwows and they, they weren't really, we weren't really allowed to go to such things. The elder people would go, but they didn't want to teach the younger people, somehow, they weren't allowed to let us practice our culture. I learned that stuff when I came down here after I recovered from alcohol. I had to learn about my own culture and other cultures . . . I'd often wonder as I was growing up why just my parents went to the powwow, not me, I wanted to learn the stuff when I was a kid, but I wasn't allowed to participate. Today I can, we can all, I'm not the only one that went through stuff like this; other Native Americans, depends on what tribe you were from or something. My tribe was, we weren't allowed to practice our traditions with our kids. Today I think it's a little bit different. The regalia people wear today is all new, I mean it's, [in] the old days just parents were involved. Today it's everybody's involved. When I go to a powwow here, sometimes you see the tiny tots when they go, a special dance for them. I wish I would have learned it a long time ago.

History plays a large role in the constitution of individual, ethnic, and collective identities, but not only through top-down identity politics—the process occurs in a bottom-up fashion as well.[16] There are different ways in which groups use their history to express the collective identities of the present. A shared history of oppression, scholars have found, can play a significant role in modern understandings of group membership and identity, shaping relationships with other communities and individuals. In Venezuela, David Guss found that Afro-Venezuelans highlight the parallels of their modern life experience with those of their Cimarron ancestors through contemporary festivals, ceremonies, and celebrations. In these events they focus on the tradition of dignified resistance to oppression, creating an unbroken link to the past.[17] At the same time, some communities reconceptualize histories of oppression in modern times in ways that reflect contemporary concerns. Scott Simon describes how Formosans who lived under Chinese Nationalist marshal law for forty years grew to look fondly upon the Japanese colonial rule of the island that preceded Chinese Nationalist rule.[18]

Thus, it is not surprising that the experience of oppression survived by Indigenous Americans through relations with the federal government, state governments, and individual cases of discrimination is a history that Natives index today in speaking about identity. In a discussion of Native poet Laura Tohe's work, linguistic anthropologist Anthony Webster describes how Tohe demonstrates her Native identity through the use of terms commonly associated with boarding school experiences, using the terms "Cats" and "Stomps" to indicate her membership in the generation that survived that experience.[19] Similarly, for Indigenous Americans living in cities, shared experiences in urban life contribute to one's sense of identity. In Deborah Davis Jackson's work on the pseudonymously named Midwestern town of Riverton, Michigan, Indigenous identity is in great part about the lived experience of being Native in the city. As Jackson explains, the urban elders faced racism, discrimination, and alcoholism in cities and while they do not outwardly display their Native heritage, they are Native because they have lived it: "Elder generation Anishinaabe people—those who grew up in the home communities of the early twentieth century—do not often seek their Indianness, nor do they usually express it in self-conscious ways. What they do—daily, subtly, with grace and gentle humor—is live it."[20] Supporting Jackson's conclusions, Susan Lobo explains that for San Francisco Bay Area Natives identity is about a shared history and shared values.[21]

The history that Jackson describes for urban Natives in Michigan is similar to the experiences of Natives in Chicago, who faced widespread racial discrimination against them in workplaces, in schools, and in neighborhoods.[22] Younger generations, whose parents faced discrimination both on the reservation and in cities, feel they must work harder to get involved in their Native traditions in order to enact their identity than someone born on the reservation. These younger generations explain that those born on a reservation are ascribed Native identity, while the urban Natives have to achieve it through study and performance. This younger generation must strive to learn about tribal culture, history, and language both on their own and through participation in Indigenous organizations in the city because, as Alfred and Randall describe, these things are not always taught by the elders due to the discrimination and oppression they faced in the past.

In the 1960s and 1970s there was a resurgence in Native identification; between 1970 and 1980, there was a 72 percent increase in the number of individuals who identified as American Indian/Alaskan Native on the United States census.[23] C. Matthew Snipp claims that this increase was due to political mobilization through acts of self-determination during this period, which promoted tribal culture and resurgence in American Indian/Alaskan Native ancestry through intertribal Indigenous movements in urban areas.[24] Deborah Davis Jackson describes a second possible factor in this increase; she found many participants in her study had been unaware of their Native ancestry early in their lives and began identifying as such on census forms upon learning the truth. According to Jackson's description of four accounts from second-generation Natives living in Riverton, the parents of these individuals faced high levels of discrimination in the workplace, being called names like "Indian Joe" or "Chief." While their parents had varied responses to these forms of workplace discrimination and varied ways of speaking about Indigenous identity, each of the four individuals Jackson worked with demonstrated that during the 1950s to be Native in the city was to be discriminated against, and so the parents of her interlocuters did not disclose their ancestry to them until later in their lives.[25]

The experience of being Native, as Jackson puts it—having lived it—and being able to index that experience of shared history, often of shared oppression survived, plays into urban Native identity today. In Chicago, people like Larry and Randall speak of the oppression their parents and grandparents endured and how that plays a role in shaping their own worldview and experience. Younger generations in Chicago consider their parents' lived history as part of their own identity and experience today, a phenomenon particularly true among those who have had to strike out on their own later in life to learn more about their culture and traditions.

Maintaining Ties with Reservation Communities

In 1971 J. Anthony Paredes suggested considering urban Native communities as part of a larger system with reservations.[26] Renya Ramirez further developed and theorized the concept in her 2007 work *Native Hubs*, proposing that urban Native community events and gatherings, like those found in the Santa Clara Valley Native community with which she worked, can serve as central hubs of the system Paredes suggests. According to Ramirez, Natives travel in and out of the hub spaces, from cities to reservations and the reverse. In the process, intertribal alliances are made, information is shared, and a network is formed. Ramirez further describes that this form of transnationalism—living in a United States city while continuing contact with home tribes—keeps urban Natives connected with their individual tribes and creates a sense of cultural identity.[27]

Transnationalism is practiced among other ethnic populations within the United States. Edna Viruell-Fuentes describes the different ways in which multiple generations of female Mexican immigrants engage in it while living in Detroit. First-generation women maintain contact with their family through monthly or bimonthly phone calls, by sending materials to their family in Mexico, and by purchasing homes in that country. Viruell-Fuentes explains that for these first-generation immigrants, the phone calls are the primary source of support, helping the women to feel a sense of belonging in the United States while at the same time reminding them that there are people in Mexico thinking about them. In the second generation, women gain a sense of pride in their history and a stronger sense of identity through trips to Mexico during which they learn about their heritage and identity.[28] Contact with home communities is significant in developing a sense of identity for many cultures living away from their extended families. As I noted in the previous chapter, many Chicago Natives visit their reservation one or more times each year. Some go to visit family, while others go to participate in ceremonies, vote in political elections, and/or fish, hunt, and gather foods on traditional tribal lands. On these trips, people often go along with friends from other tribes and learn about and participate in the tribal ceremonies and events of other tribes than their own. Members of this community also live for portions of their life on a reservation, and not necessarily on a reservation of which they are a tribal citizen.

At the conclusion of such visits, Chicago Natives will often bring Native items for consumption back to share in Chicago. Consumption has long been recognized as a feature of identity performance within the social sciences.[29] Indeed, consuming certain types of food is a way of identifying who you are and who you are not; culinary choices mark ethnicity and create distinctions between self and other.[30] At the senior lunches I observed between 2007 and 2014, seniors highly praised those meals that incorporated Native foods, such as venison, bison, squash, beans, corn, hominy, walleye, berries and wild rice, along with frybread.[31] At the first senior lunch in the American Indian Center's new Albany Park location, hosted in April of 2019, the meal consisted of several foods centered on Indigenous traditions. This meal included a three sisters' vegetable side dish of mixed corn, green beans, and zucchini squash and a dessert made up of mixed berry crisp, sweetened with Splenda for those conscious of their sugar intake. Food is a cultural connector in this context. In the case of those attending senior lunches, meals featuring Native food items that were not part of their own ancestors' diets are still seen as connecting them to their Indigenous American ancestry. Consuming the traditional foods of a tribe that is not one's own not only serves to connect an individual to their Indigenous American ancestry but further binds individuals of a diverse set of Indigenous American tribes together in Chicago as a community.

In addition to obtaining Native foods from the reservations for community meals, Chicago Native community members bring back plants and Native medicines for use in the city space. Cedar is brought for tea, sage for smudging, and plant seeds and saplings from reservation lands to grow in Chicago soil. In 2015 members of the center planted eight-hundred-year-old seeds found on an archaeological site in Menominee territory in the garden space outside of the building on Wilson Avenue. The squash produced was served and shared with the larger community later that fall at the Giving Thanks Feast. Native plants, then, are not only growing between the cracks of the pavement, as Rosanna described in her statement at the beginning of this chapter; they are also planted and cultivated in dedicated city spaces for Native gardens and tended by community members.

The road between the reservation and the city is traveled both ways. Some tribes also bring services to the city. In Chicago, a direct and constant relationship with the reservation is seen in the relations between the Chicago Ho-Chunk and the Wisconsin Ho-Chunk government. The Ho-Chunk Nation of Wisconsin set up an office in Chicago in 1993, the Ho-Chunk Nation Urban Branch Office.[32] The office provides Ho-Chunk members with government services, such as tribal loans for housing and education, as well as health and social services. Its goal is to strengthen the link between the Wisconsin tribe and their relatives in Chicago. A meeting is held each month, at which the tribal legislators and Chicago Ho-Chunk share a prayer and a meal and discuss new legislation and events happening in the Ho-Chunk government. This opening of the Ho-Chunk office shows the importance of the associations being maintained between urban and reservation tribal members.[33] The American Indian Center maintains a close relationship with several of the local tribes, including the Menominee and the Potawatomi tribes, which offer both financial and personnel support for some of the center's programming.

Performance

I had been volunteering daily at the American Indian Center for six months, answering phones in reception, working with the weekly food pantry, assisting in the cooking and serving of the senior lunch, and helping with preparations for the center's fifty-ninth annual Chicago Powwow, when I poked my head into Rebecca's office to tell her I was on the way home for the day and said "goodbye." Exasperated, Rebecca stopped me as I began to turn to leave, saying: "Meg, we do not say goodbye, we say see you." Rebecca explained that "goodbye" implies finality, and that even when someone passes away, it is customary to say "see you" rather than "goodbye." Through calling my attention to a daily faux pas after months of volunteering at the center, Rebecca was inviting me to become more involved in the community as an insider rather than an outsider. One of the many ways in which people identify themselves as members of a group is through performance.

According to anthropologist and sociologist Edward H. Spicer,

Native identity is a flexible category, based not so much upon an association with land or the practice of tradition as it is on the ideas and feelings about the various events that people have shared together and lived through: "Being an Indian means participating in the Indian realm of meaning regarding these events which both Indians and whites have experienced . . . meanings which make the real difference between Indians and others."[34] In Native Chicago, performances of Native identity go beyond blood and shared history to include speaking a Native language and participating in rituals and other events.

Anthropologist Jessica Cattelino explains that members of the Seminole Nation see the loss of language as equating to a loss of culture.[35] Similarly, the ability to speak Native languages was a primary aspect that the film *Red Cry* turned to in describing urban Natives as not knowing their culture. Rebecca, a fifty-three-year-old Odawa/Omaha woman, describes how in the past, Chicago community members would continue to use their Native languages in conversation. However, echoing Alfred earlier in this chapter, Rebecca noted that parents did not pass Native languages down to their children, fearing that the latter would be taken away:

REBECCA: My dad would talk, there were several people in the community that would talk, Agnes, and some of the other ones that would, Arlene's mom, she said oh we all used to speak Ojibwe with your dad and we'd all be laughing. They said that's when we would really get to speak our language was when we all got together was when they were all at the Indian Center. So I never realized that. I knew when we went back home to Canada that everybody up there that was the first language. And they'd use English occasionally. But he said he didn't want me to learn because everyone, it seemed like everyone was scared they were going to take the kids away and make us all go to boarding school.

Today the majority of Chicago Natives speak English as a first language, although some community members do know Native languages. Participants in this study described having knowledge of or having a family member with knowledge of Diné, Choctaw, Lakota, and several dialects of Ojibwe and Pueblo. At the same time, few could claim fluency, with most participants knowing only a few words of these languages. This paucity of fluent speakers in Chicago stands in contrast to the situation on the reservations, some of which have dedicated Native language classes and schools for children that have no direct counterpart in the city.[36] In an effort to remedy this state of affairs, language-learning groups have cropped up throughout the city; meanwhile, the youth program at the American Indian Center strives to teach some Native words to younger generations. An Ojibwe language class began in Chicago in January 2015. As described to me by one participant in this class, the students include members not only of Ojibwe-speaking-Nations but also of other tribes. Similar to the consumption of Native foods described above, there is a great interest in learning about and participating in Native cultural traditions and activities in the city space as a way not only of connecting with one's individual ancestry but also of engaging in the intertribal community and Indigenous American culture more broadly.

Participation in spiritual and ritual events constitutes a performance of Native identity. Based upon his ethnographic and survey research, anthropologist Eli Suzukovich finds that Chicago Natives participate in a wide range of religious practices and belief systems in the city, including Traditional beliefs (Tribal belief systems, Native American Church, Midewiwin, Big Drum, and Longhouse), Christian beliefs (Catholic, Protestant, Episcopalian, Born Again Christian, and Seventh Day Adventist), and in mixed religious practices that combine these Traditional and Christian systems. Spiritual events are common, and include sweat lodges, morning prayers, naming ceremonies, healing ceremonies, pipe ceremonies, drum feasts, sunrise ceremonies, wakes, funeral celebrations, and Sunday masses. However, as Suzukovich explains, many of these practices are unseen, that is, they exist as personal or intimate performances rather than public ones.[37] These events are often held within homes and are announced via word of mouth.

Individual identities are negotiated through discursive interactions and performances. One may perform an identity, but its confirmation relies upon the acknowledgment of one's interlocutors.[38] After one senior lunch in the summer of 2013, Roy stopped by the table where other volunteers and I were eating to chat for a few minutes when he noticed a flyer inviting people to attend a sweat lodge in one of the northwestern suburbs. He commented that this flyer was not right, adding that the traditional way was to spread news of the event via word of mouth. Participation in the event, then, is not the only performance of identity: so too is the way in which the news is spread. Roy's contestation of this sweat lodge host's performance of Native identity demonstrates that there is pressure in the city to enact Native identity in a certain way. Roy was engaging in boundary maintenance, just as the elder woman was doing after that senior lunch when she challenged the newcomer who was attempting to sell Native artifacts' claim to Native heritage.

Other performances of Native identity in Chicago include participating in powwows, dancing, drumming, storytelling, and behaving in what are described as Native ways. Powwows are a significant aspect of urban Native life. Not only do members of Chicago's Native community host several powwows throughout the year, some also follow the powwow trail—attending, dancing, drumming, and selling food and crafts in powwows across the United States and Canada. Telling stories is another activity Chicago Natives described to me as a way of enacting their Native identity and passing culture and tradition on to their children. Lastly, behaving in a Native way was described as important to Native identity. Behaviors commonly referred to as tied to Native traditions included sharing what you have with others, respecting women, and having a reverence for the earth. For example, Rosanna described holding a worldview that is distinctly Native, one that is made up of each of these factors— from carrying the knowledge of a shared history of oppression to showing reverence and respect for the earth and for one another.

Being Native in the City Space

Natives living in cities like Chicago are performing and negotiating their Native identity in a space surrounded by people representing a diverse array of cultural and ethnic backgrounds. Living in this space, people learn to balance their identity. Urban Natives adopt cultural items and values of city life while retaining Native values and cultural ways. Roy, a thirty-five-year-old Oglala Sioux/Navajo man, described what it was like growing up Native in the city:

> ROY: Different from other, different in a sense from, from an outsider, from well, two perspectives. One perspective inside, one outside. So more of perspective from the inside, so just trying to balance city life and sort of Indian life if you may.
>
> MEG: So, what exactly does that mean?
>
> ROY: Well, I mean like being a part of I would say mainstream in a sense. And then be more of underground with what I've been taught in a sense from my tribal culture, 'cause it's . . . there are, there are differences, and there are similarities, so just trying to find a balance between both mainstream and my tribal cultures if you may.

While Roy speaks of managing his identity, aiming to strike a balance between his Native identity and his urban life, community elders are concerned that the younger generations are not learning from the older ones. It appears to be a perennial problem in many contexts worldwide, where older generations see changes in youth behavior as indicative of culture loss. For instance, Michael Herzfeld finds in his work with artisan apprentices in Greece that older generations view taking up aspects of modern life as equivalent to losing one's cultural identity.[39] The younger generations, of which Roy is a part, explain that they do follow their Native traditions; at the same time, they incorporate some aspects of urban life into their identities. Roy, for instance, drums, participates in powwows and traditional ceremonies, visits and has lived on reservations, but he is also an avid member of online communities, plays video games, and enjoys watching Hollywood blockbusters.

Urban Natives are involved in a variety of communities outside of Native life, including work, school, volunteer organizations, neighborhoods, churches, and sports. In the city space, people adopt cultural items and values from these non-Native spheres of life while retaining Native values and cultural ways.[40]

Concepts of identity change over time. As James Clifford highlights in his discussion of the Mashpee court case, all cultures change—no one group is static for all of time, and this fact is especially true for cultures that are changing in an environment of domination.[41] In the context of communities that are separate from their homeland, identities can be flexible and overlapping. Dalia Abdelhady's work describes the different ways in which Lebanese immigrants in Montreal, Paris, and New York belong to three separate communities: their host country, the diasporic community within their host country, and the Lebanese immigrant communities throughout the world. Abdelhady shows that immigrants do not have a singular membership in any one community; rather, there are ways of participating in multiple separate and fragmented communities while retaining dedication to Lebanese autonomy.[42]

Like the Lebanese in Abdelhady's discussion, Chicago Natives are managing their Native identity in a diverse locale through balance. New cultural forms are adapted to urban life, as the traditional practices may not function in the urban setting as they would on a reservation. Traditions and identities evolve with time and in place, and younger generations of Chicago Natives are developing and negotiating their own ways of managing their Native identity in the urban space.

Relationships with Non-Natives

Part of the balance that Roy speaks of achieving is done within interactions with non-Natives. In an interview, Mary, a fifty-seven-year-old Menominee woman, described being dismayed by an acquaintance's assumptions after telling this person about a planned trip to the Menominee reservation:

MARY: She's like oh, the reservation, are there teepees on there? I'm like, Alice, are you talking to me or what? I had to laugh, I'm like, I told Alice later I was going to say I can't believe you asked me that question when you're like a smart person. Of course there's no fucking teepees on there. It's like small town living, I told her, kind of like towns gathered together around the lake, it's not, there's no teepees unless you make a fake one in your driveway or something. Yes, really? So I mean sometimes that surprises me and then she, I think when she said it, she was embarrassed, I said Alice that would be like me thinking oh, you're Mexican, do you have like a dirt floor house, or what. She was like, oh yeah. So I didn't, I did answer her and I showed her pictures you know where my mom lives and then around the lake and everything and how beautiful it is and it's all just small-town living. I said you wouldn't be able to survive there unless you have a car you know or a good truck in the winter. So I think that's a challenge because I really, it's a stereotype kind of thing and it, it happened to me a lot when I was a nurse, a manager too.

What occurred in Mary's interaction is not uncommon. In the week before the American Indian Center's sixty-first annual powwow, community members were excited by publicity for the event that was made possible by the local news channel WGN picking up the story and inviting dancers and drummers to perform for a segment of their morning broadcast. In this segment, which aired on September 10, 2014, one newscaster described the event as the community honoring the "Relocation Act of the 1950s" and another newscaster later referred to Chicago Natives as though they were all members of a single tribe. These occasions of misunderstanding represent pressures from non-Natives on contemporary definitions of Native identity. Yet, these types of interactions are spaces in which Chicago Natives choose to either ignore or push back against stereotypes or misunderstandings and define Native culture, traditions, history, and identity in the contemporary context.

In *Indians in Unexpected Places* Philip Deloria describes how many non-Native Americans do not expect to find Natives living in urban centers. Deloria explains that this is because urban Natives do not match up with the expectations non-Natives have of who Indigenous American peoples are.[43] In the collective conscious-ness of most Americans, Native Americans are thought of not as an urban populace but as members of a reservation community. Oftentimes, non-Natives are not aware of the large Native popula-tion in Chicago. Community organizers see this as one of the larg-est challenges faced by the Native community, as it hinders their ability to gain access to financial resources to support programs. Joshua, a community organizer, explained:

> JOSHUA: We're just an invisible part of Chicago's community, and we need to become more visible. And I think one of the say-ings that the organization that I belong to is making the invisible visible . . . I think that the mayor's office needs to do something to recognize Indian people. I think Indian people need to make them more aware of us by having a big powwow downtown in Grant Park or something, just to show we're here. [sixty-four-year-old White Earth Chippewa man]

Two weeks after my interview with Joshua, at a meeting of the Coa-lition of Chicago American Indian Community Organizations—the group Joshua spoke of—organizers described the frustrations they faced as not-for-profit organizations seeking funding. One participant of this meeting described how, in a rejection explana-tion from a grant application her organization received, the funder noted that they had already supported a Native program located in the Southwestern United States. The organizer asked those of us in attendance at the meeting to consider whether any funder would offer this same explanation to a Black or a Latinx organiza-tion. The invisibility of urban Native populations to non-Natives is widespread, despite the fact that most Natives reside in urban areas, and has been documented in Chicago's Native community in previ-ous scholarship that focuses on the community's marginalization.[44]

My point here is not to essentialize all non-Natives as though they are unaware of the Native population of the city and have no clue about Native history or contemporary Native culture, but to note that the majority of Chicago's inhabitants are unaware that the city is home to the eighth largest Native population in the United States, and that many Natives feel they have to educate those they encounter in the city who hold stereotypes of Natives. Both Mary's interaction with her friend and the coalition's discussion of trying to increase the visibility of the community demonstrate the ways in which Chicago Natives perform acts of politics of identity, challenging widely held stereotypes about who and where Native people are today.

A Community of Survival

At the annual American Indian Center Giving Thanks Feast in November of 2013, a community elder and founding member of the center led the community in prayer before the meal began. In her welcoming address, she stated that she was thankful for the survival of Native communities—from surviving the first Thanksgiving through surviving as an urban Native community today. This elder's sentiments, Rosanna's statement quoted in the introduction to this chapter, and the comments of Elmer on Native peoples representing cultures of survival described in the previous chapter are examples of how multiple generations of Chicago Natives take pride in their and their ancestors' accomplishments in being able to survive centuries of struggles against colonialism, oppression, and attempts of assimilation.

Chicago's Native community is diverse, being made up of tribes from across the United States and Canada. Maintaining individual tribal identities and contact with tribes is important to Chicago Natives, and the relationship between the city and the reservation is one that is actively maintained by both the urban and reservation Natives. One of the largest support systems for Natives in Chicago is the network of relationships between Natives in the city, supported in great part by organizations supporting intertribal Native community and traditions. These include the American Indian

Center of Chicago, the Saint Kateri Center (a now Catholic organization, formerly known as the Anawim Center), Saint Augustine's Center, the Mitchell Museum of the American Indian, the American Indian Association of Illinois, the California Manpower Consortium, and American Indian Health Service of Chicago.[45]

The American Indian Center of Chicago is described by many members of the community as the flagship Native institution; this is because it is the first organization most people, both Native and non-Native, come across when searching out Natives in the city. The American Indian Center of Chicago is the oldest center of its kind in the nation. As described in the introductory chapter, in 1953 community members, some of whom had been involved in developing previous organizations in Chicago and others who were new to the city, established the All Tribes American Indian Center, with an emphasis on the first two words in the name. Although supported by the Bureau of Indian Affairs, the center from its early years was a Native-run organization. From its beginnings as a social gathering place, over the years it developed a social service function and became central to the identity of the Chicago Native community. For example, as one participant in the 1980s Chicago American Indian Oral History Pilot Project explained in her interview, she likely would have left the city had she not found the center due to the loneliness she faced in the city.[46] Intertribal alliances in cities across the United States first developed to combat such loneliness.[47] Natives living in Chicago, as well as in Rochester and the California Bay Area, explain that it is easier to maintain Native identity through participation in intertribal Native organizations in the city because they promote cultural values and traditions.[48]

The American Indian Center is central to many people's stories about their lives growing up in Native Chicago. While some people intermittently visit the center on holidays, for powwows, and for ceremonies, others are involved in its day-to-day programs. Rebecca is a self-proclaimed "center baby." Her parents met at the center, held their wedding reception and her baby shower there, and Rebecca has been involved in the center for most of her life.

She recalled going to powwows at two of the center's (at the time of this interview) three locations while growing up in one of the city's suburbs:

REBECCA: I don't remember the first center. I remember the second one over on Sheridan Road and going upstairs and they had big powwows when we had monthly powwows, there were like eight, nine drums set up. We had the Chippewa Drum and Menomonie Drum and Winnebago Drum, Family Drums, Sioux Drum, Southern Style Wipponka Drum, and a lot of people danced. It was, the rooms were just full. [fifty-three-year-old Odawa/Omaha woman]

The center brought people from tribes across the United States together and was a place where community members now in their middle age recall growing up.

Arlene, a sixty-three-year-old Ojibwe/Odawa woman who grew up in the city, recalled going to each of the locales the center has stood in over the past sixty years:

ARLENE: My mom used to bring us to powwows. I went, I remember going to powwows on LaSalle. Now that was a long time ago. That was in the '50s and I remember going up there, my mom used to take us. That was a long time ago. But I remember going there. It was, I think that was the first Indian Center that was in Chicago. They moved from LaSalle to I think the next one was on Sheridan and Broadway. It was on the corner there. No, it was on Sheridan and Broadway. There was an Indian Center there. It's gone now. There's a gas station there now. But there was another, there was an Indian Center there, and then from there I think they moved over here.

In addition to going to powwows as a child, Arlene "hung out" at the center as a teen, met her ex-husband in those teenage years, and now volunteers at the center each week.

Through these intertribal networks, many Natives meet future spouses from other tribes. Gerard, a forty-four-year-old Choctaw/ Navajo man, laughingly spoke of how he has to often explain his mixed-Native ancestry to people:

GERARD: My mom's from Mississippi, Choctaw, and my dad's from New Mexico and they came here through the relocation, brought them to Chicago. They were both placed, I always get this, you know they're like the people who know tribes and the geographical regions of the tribes and they're like how did you become Choctaw Navajo, they're two different parts of the country, it's because of relocation and because my parents were placed in the same neighborhood.

The relocation program brought Natives from across the United States together. Not only did people partner with citizens of other tribes, but they also shared traditions and practices in the urban space, as is also occurring in the Santa Clara Valley.[49] Diane, a twenty-seven-year-old Arikara/Omaha/Odawa woman, explained that one of the great things about Native life in a city is that they learn about other Native cultures:

DIANE: Growing up, one advantage is here in the city is you learn not only your ways, is you learn a whole bunch of tribes' ways, like I know a lot of Navajo ways or Ho-Chunk ways, or Potawatomi, Menominee ways that I know there's a lot of different ways to do things, so I've learned some of the different, so if I go to travel to different areas, I kind of know what you can and can't do when you're over there.

For Diane, knowing different ways has been useful as she and her family travel throughout the year. They visit Native communities for powwows and other events around the United States and Canada, and she feels better prepared to participate in events at each site than she would have only knowing her own tribes' cultures.

Though the name has changed, the center activities reflect its initial name, All-Indian. Steven explained in an interview on what it meant to be Native in Chicago:

STEVEN: In Chicago, is that you're, you're not just from your tribe, there's so many different tribes here in the city that you're not, it doesn't matter what tribe you are. You're still an Indian. Once you come to the center, we're all Indians here and it doesn't matter what Indian you are or what you are. We're all united as the Indians in Chicago, you know what I mean, it's, we're all one type of Indian. Where you can't say oh well, I belong to this tribe, I belong to that tribe. [sixty-one-year-old Seneca man]

Steven's sentiments are not shared by everyone. There are members of some of the older generations who choose not to participate in the center because they do not feel that the people they could meet at the center are their people. One particular area of contention in recent history was the American Indian Center's association and partnership with the Chicago Blackhawks—a National Hockey team that uses Native imagery. The center recently ended its partnership with the organization and released a statement indicating that they would in the future avoid ties with any organization perpetuating harmful stereotypes.[50]

The Native community of Chicago is not one single community that exists without dispute. However, Veronica explained that the community comes together when it is needed:

VERONICA: It's just that when things occur to us, we try to pull together as a community or as a group, or as a family to help each other out. Like if someone's gets, one time there was somebody that had a fire in their apartment, so we were going around getting things that they needed to set up and somebody was helping them find an apartment. You know we try to be there to help when we know somebody is in trouble or needs some kind of assistance. We try to be there and do what we can. Sometimes if it's not physically possible, at least we try to encourage them to, to hang in there until times get better. And of course you know we have our, when someone dies in the community, we have their memorial service. [San Juan Pueblo/Old Laguna Pueblo elder, age not disclosed]

While people like Steven and Veronica both speak of coming together, there are many instances where divisions can be seen.

Chicago's Native organizations are trying to work together today to find more funding to support community programs, but infighting in recent years has detracted from their ability to do so. Larry, a leader of one organization, explained:

LARRY: They're not united. They're going through a process now with a lot of the agencies of uniting and being a united front politically. There's been a whole strategic planning over the last year. They've gotten further along with that than they ever have, which is a great sign, so I think a lot of it is newer people coming on board that are leaders, wanting to change. You still have some infighting. [fifty-three-year-old Covelo man]

Chicago's Native community is an intertribal one, made up of smaller networks of people. As with all communities, there are disputes from time to time, but the community pulls together in times of need, as they did for the healing circle that followed the Truth Tour event in April of 2013.

Members of Chicago's Native community articulate a story of survival when reflecting upon the Urban Indian Relocation Program and on the longer history of Natives in relation to European settlers. Native identity in the city is deeply rooted in history and politics, while performed and negotiated in the present. Chicago Natives factor blood, histories of oppression, contact with reservation communities, language, food, religious beliefs, behaviors, and relationships with non-Natives into their concepts of identity.

Today, Chicago's Native community does not represent a cohesive singular unit; rather, it is a network of people who at times are at odds with one another, and at other times come together. Urban Natives identify both with individual tribes and as members of an intertribal Indigenous community in which members practice traditions, learn languages, and eat foods that historically belonged to a variety of tribes. This sharing of Native traditions in the urban space works not only to bind the community together as an ethnic enclave in the city space but also to connect individuals to a broader Indigenous American history and identity. Now that I have briefly sketched out Chicago's Native community, in the next chapter I begin to describe diabetes in Native populations and in humanity more broadly.

3

Diabetes among Indigenous Americans

O ld invoices, handwritten notes, and crumpled paper napkins were strewn across the desk between us as Steven talked about his experiences with diabetes. A sixty-one-year-old Seneca man who moved from the Tonawanda Reservation in upstate New York to Chicago in 1979, Steven is a slender man with ear-length, jet-black hair and glasses. While it is hard to imagine Steven at a larger size, he shared that at the time of his diagnosis with diabetes fifteen years earlier he was seventy-five pounds heavier. His weight loss helped him to take control of diabetes, a control, he explained, that requires knowledge and self-discipline. Upon his diagnosis, Steven immediately quit drinking alcohol and smoking cigarettes, and over time learned how certain foods and activities affected his blood glucose control. Half an hour into our interview Steven's wife, Susan, poked her head into this office on the lower level of the American Indian Center to see if we were done, jesting that Steven likes to talk and I should stop him if he is going on too long. Steven retorted that he never gets to talk at home, and is going to use this opportunity as he pleases. After Susan left, laughing along with us at his reply, we returned to our conversation on diabetes and its causes. While describing the factors that can lead to diabetes, Steven noted that Natives have particularly high rates of the disease. I asked him to elaborate on why he thinks that is the case.

STEVEN: This is a personal view of mine. I think that the way that the Native American people have been susceptible—to live the white man's way, to live the way the white man lives and to eat the white man's food . . . few hundred years ago, there was no such thing as smallpox, there was no diseases here until the white man came across this ocean and brought them with him. The Indians never had no problems with any of that thing or anything like that. Common colds and stuff like that maybe, but nothing as rampant as these [referring to smallpox and diabetes].

In this chapter we take a step back both in time and in perspective to look at the history of diabetes in extant human records and in Native American populations. While diabetes is relatively new to Native North Americans, it has a long history in other parts of the world, having affected humans for thousands of years.[1] While it was known to exist in Old World contexts for millennia, diagnoses of diabetes among the Indigenous peoples of North America were rare prior to the mid-twentieth century.[2] Since that time the rate of diabetes has rapidly grown in these populations, as it simultaneously rose in other indigenous contexts worldwide.[3] In the United States, Indigenous peoples have the highest rates of diabetes when compared with other ethnic groups. According to 2020 CDC estimates, 14.7 percent of Indigenous American adults are living with diabetes, compared to 12.5 percent of Hispanics, 11.7 percent of Non-Hispanic Blacks, 9.2 percent of Asian Americans, and 7.5 percent of Non-Hispanic Whites. Within Native populations, the rates of diabetes vary by tribe. In 2017 the CDC estimated that as low as 5.5 percent of the Alaskan Native population was living with diabetes, while some Southwestern nations had a rate as high as 22.2 percent among adults.[4] Today Indigenous Americans not only have some of the highest rates of diabetes but are developing the condition earlier in life and have higher rates of related complications when compared with other ethnic populations in the United States.[5]

My aim in this chapter is to provide a brief overview of diabetes. I begin by providing a brief and partial history of this disease, relying on extant written records of what has been interpreted as early cases of the condition. I contextualize these early accounts by describing the features of the ancient Greco-Roman medical model under which many of these accounts were written. I include this history both to give readers a sense of the long history of diabetes in humans generally in contrast to the very recent development of diabetes cases in specifically Indigenous American populations, and to compare features of historical models of diabetes to contemporary biomedical understandings of the disease. While there are other accounts of diabetes in early human history in the Old World, I focus primarily on Greco-Roman records because the contemporary biomedical model of the condition that is most often utilized by the participants of this study is built upon them. After looking at the history of diabetes from antiquity through the development of insulin therapy, I turn to modern definitions of diabetes, using interview excerpts and published biomedical materials to explore the contemporary biomedical model. Finally, I describe the relatively recent diabetes epidemic in Indigenous American populations and review biomedical explanations for why people develop diabetes, with a particular focus on reasons for why Native Americans are affected at such high rates today. I argue that the contemporary diabetes epidemic among Indigenous Americans was engendered by colonial policies. As foreshadowed by Steven's description, there are local definitions and explanations for diabetes in Native communities that both mirror and diverge from the biomedical explanations explored in this chapter; these are the focus of chapters 4 and 5.

A Brief History of Diabetes in the Western World

Diabetes existed in Old World contexts more than three millennia ago.[6] While the earliest extant accounts of diabetes date back thirty-five hundred years, it is possible that premodern hominin species experienced the condition during earlier periods in history for which we do not have written evidence. For instance, scholars have found that Neanderthals carried a gene that today is associated with the development of type 2 diabetes.[7] The experience of diabetes in prehistory and antiquity would have been very different from the diabetes we know now—today physicians recognize multiple manifestations of the disease and there are therapies to manage the condition, whereas diabetes in ancient texts is described as a singular condition classified with other fatal diseases.

Medical historians identify the existence of diabetes in antiquity based upon descriptions of symptoms commonly linked to the condition—polyuria and polydipsia, or frequent urination and excessive thirst. Entries in the Papyrus Ebers, written around 1500 BCE in Egypt, describe several remedies and ointments for treating polyuria.[8] Though Hippocrates is described as not studying diseases he could not effectively treat, there are some indirect references to what is thought to be diabetes in the Hippocratic Corpus, specifically descriptions of polyuria.[9] Despite these early references, the condition known today as diabetes was not commonly referred to using that label until several centuries after Hippocrates's lifetime. There is some dispute over who was first to coin the term "diabetes," which in ancient Greek translates to "siphon." While some historians of the disease ascribe the term to Demetrius of Apamea, others credit Aretæus of Cappadocia with its invention.[10]

While Aretæus may or may not be responsible for the naming of diabetes, he is credited with having written the most complete description of the disease in antiquity.[11] Aretæus describes the application of the term diabetes to this condition: "It seems to me that the epithet Diabetes has been assigned from the disorder being something like passing of water by a siphon, since the liquid does not remain in the body, but makes use of the patient to escape as it would by a bridge."[12] According to Aretæus, for those who have developed diabetes, the body acts as a bridge, channel, or ladder for water to pass through. Aretæus notes the similarity of the disease to the effects of a bite from the dispas snake, a bite that was fabled to engender a great thirst in the person bitten.

Aretæus's description of diabetes is focused on the outward physical effects it has on the affected individual's body. Here, diabetes does not immediately attack and destroy the human body; rather, it slowly establishes its presence. As the disease progresses, the symptoms worsen: "Life too is odious and painful, the thirst is ungovernable, and the copious potations are more than equaled by the profuse urinary discharge; for more urine flows away, and it is impossible to put any restraint to the patient's drinking or making water. For if he stop for a very brief period, and leave off drinking, the mouth becomes parched, the body dry; the bowels seem on fire, he is wretched and uneasy, and soon dies, tormented with burning thirst."[13] Furthermore, Aretæus asks, "How indeed could the making of water be stopped, or what sense of modesty is paramount to pain? But if he continue to place restraint on himself for a short time, then loins, testicles, and ischia swell, and when he relaxes, he discharges a vastly profuse quantity of water, and the swelling subsides, for the superfluity passes by the bladder."[14] In reading Aretæus's description we become privy to the experience of diabetes in antiquity—dry mouth, frequent urination, and great discomfort. The most thorough account and definition of the disease in antiquity, Aretæus's classification was not revised in western Europe until the eighteenth century.[15]

Evidence of diabetes has been found throughout the Old World in early history, far outside the European continent. In the Hindu world, one finds a disease described in the Ayurveda as being indicated through the signs of sweet or honey urine, phlegm, and sweat.[16] Between fourteen hundred and two thousand years ago, Charaka, Sushruta, and Vagbhata described the sweetness of urine in some individuals, almost one thousand years before their European counterparts did, by noting the attraction of ants to the urine of those afflicted with this ailment.[17] In the third and fourth centuries CE, Chinese physician Tchang-Thoug-King noted that dogs were attracted to the urine of those who had a malady of thirst.[18] In the tenth century CE the renowned Arab physician Avicenna, like Aretæus, wrote a detailed account of the symptoms and progression of diabetes.[19]

Worldwide, diabetes was an acute and fatal disease until the early twentieth century. As noted above, its definition in Western medicine did not significantly change between Aretæus's lifetime in the first century CE and the eighteenth century. During this expanse of time, treatment for the condition aimed to minimize symptoms and ease pain before death.[20] In the early twentieth century, the understanding of and care for diabetes transitioned to a different level, with the development of insulin therapy.

Treating Diabetes in the Twentieth Century

In 1921 diabetes shifted from an acute disease to a chronic condition with the successful extraction and purification of insulin for injection in humans.[21] This breakthrough came after several decades of research that determined the role of insulin in living organisms. The processes of the science behind this development, of course, are more complicated than this brief history shows. Science and technology studies scholars Bruno Latour, Steven Woolgar, Andrew Pickering, and Karin Knorr Cetina show that the work done in laboratories is a long and complicated process of negotiation between scientists and their objects of study.[22] Highlighting some of the key events here, I recognize that years of failed experiments and running into dead ends also played a significant role in shaping the biomedical model of diabetes today. To situate this history of insulin therapy development, I first describe the medical model under which it was developed, namely, biomedicine.

As a practice, biomedicine was established as the principal medical practice in the West over the decades between the turn of the twentieth century and the end of World War II.[23] Biomedicine is not one singular practice. Rather, it is shaped by and enmeshed in the local contexts in which it is practiced.[24] Though its practice is situated within local spaces, there are features of biomedicine that bind it together across these spaces. Globally, biomedicine is reliant upon the standardization of bodies in order to understand what constitutes disease and well-being. In this system, norms are created using statistical data—and scholars note that individual corporeal bodies rarely meet these expected standards.[25] Where Greek and Roman physicians sought to locate the causes of diseases within organs, biomedicine increasingly focuses on locating disease at some of the smallest levels within the body—genes, cells, and molecules—and is dependent upon science and technology to make these human interiors visible.[26] In their work, anthropologists Margaret Lock and Vinh-Kim Nguyen demonstrate how this relationship with science, biology, and technology works to legitimate biomedicine and its use on a global scale.[27]

Understandings of diabetes transitioned along with the changes in the medical system. In antiquity the patient's symptoms were central to the definition of diabetes, which was thought to be located in the bladder or kidneys. By the late nineteenth century, scientists began to look deeper within the human body to understand the cause of the disease, no longer defining the condition primarily by the symptoms of polyuria and polydipsia. In the nineteenth century French scientists Joseph Freiherr von Mering and Oskar Minkowski learned that removing the pancreas of a dog resulted in the dog displaying diabetes symptoms. Eugene Opie found in 1901 that the pancreas's islet cells, first noted and described by Paul Langerhans in the nineteenth century, showed lesions in patients with diabetes. By 1913 Sir Edward Albert Sharpey-Schäfer and Jean de Meyer had independently referred to the hormone secreted by the islets of Langerhans as "insuline." Each hypothesized that a disturbance in the production of this hormone would lead to diabetes. In 1916 Sharpey-Schäfer suggested that the islets of the Beta cells in the pancreas secrete insulin. By 1916, then, scientists aimed to find a way to reintroduce insulin to the diabetic patient as a possible means of managing diabetes.[28]

Finding a way to do so involved a long process of trial and error. Fredrick Grant Banting and John James Rickard Macleod, along with their student assistants Charles Herbert Best and James Bertram Collip, first successfully extracted insulin for use in lowering the blood glucose of a person with diabetes in 1921.[29] Banting and Macleod won the 1923 Nobel Prize in Physiology or Medicine for this work and each shared half of their prize monies with their student assistants.[30] The patent for insulin was given to the University of Toronto for a few dollars.[31] In the 1920s the pharmaceutical company Eli Lilly and the university took up role of the mass producers of insulin, which in its early years was extracted from pigs and cattle. Today most insulin in the United States is recombinant human insulin.

Understandings of diabetes today are built upon this history of diabetes in human populations, forming a palimpsest over the descriptions of Aretæus and the studies of Sharpey-Schäfer. In the next section I look at contemporary definitions of the disease offered in biomedical publications and by biomedically trained research participants, and show how this development of insulin therapy spurred further refinements and divisions in the biomedical model of diabetes.

Defining Diabetes Today

A mesh hamper filled with cicadae rested on the long buffet table in Laura's office, their song providing a backdrop to our discussion. Having worked as a nurse in Chicago's Native community for more than a decade, Laura is involved in a wide range of projects in the community—from planting a Native food and medicine garden and hosting traditional healers and spiritual leaders for weekend events to helping members of the community manage chronic condition care. Later this afternoon she would be teaching youth at the American Indian Center about the seventeen-year lifecycle of cicadae. After two weeks of shadowing Laura in her daily routine (during my first stint of research in 2007), we sat down to discuss diabetes care in the community. Laura earned a bachelor's degree in nursing in the late 1990s after working as a registered nurse since 1980. In addition to her training in the biomedical field of nursing, Laura took courses in Ayurvedic and Chinese medicine and worked with Native American medicine men from across the Midwestern United States. In response to my question "what is diabetes," Laura defined the condition by describing its physiological traits, noting that it can lead to additional health concerns; she also mentioned local explanations for its cause in Native populations:

LAURA: We call diabetes, whether it's type one or type two, we still call it diabetes but they're two very, very different things. They happen to both end up with high blood sugar and they both happen to, can lead to a lot of the same chronic illnesses such as kidney failure, and high blood pressure, and eye problems and that kind of thing. But I think that they're two different things. So there is that, physiological part. But I once met a Ho-Chunk man who felt that diabetes was a conspiracy by the U.S. government. He was very serious about this. He felt that the government had poisoned his people a long time ago and it was now coming out. And I have to say I didn't totally disagree with him. [fifty-five-year-old non-Native nurse]

I learned within a few short weeks of beginning this research in the summer of 2007 that interviewees found the question "What is diabetes?" far more difficult to answer than I had anticipated. Participants with and without biomedical training had a hard time developing and organizing a description of what they knew as diabetes. Laura's definition stands out from other definitions offered by biomedical providers I spoke with and from those found in biomedical publications in her inclusion of this man's idea that diabetes in Native populations is a conspiracy of the United States government.

The American Diabetes Association defines diabetes as "a group of metabolic diseases characterized by hyperglycemia resulting from defects in insulin secretion, insulin action, or both. The chronic hyperglycemia of diabetes is associated with long-term damage, dysfunction, and failure of different organs, especially the eyes, kidneys, nerves, heart, and blood vessel."[32] Of the thirteen biomedical providers I spoke with, eleven providers' definitions of the condition factored in hyperglycemia, or high blood glucose levels. Additionally, biomedical providers focused on diabetes as a failure, inability, or malfunction in the body's capability to break down and metabolize food:

LAURA: The body's endocrine system does not function in the appropriate manner to keep, in particular, blood sugars in a normal range.

JANICE: Diabetes I would have to say it's the inability of the body to . . . metabolize glucose levels. It's when the blood sugars in the body are, are [more] elevated than normal. [thirty-year-old Ojibwe nurse]

Providers describe diabetes as an insufficient amount of insulin, referring specifically to the endocrine system and metabolism. According to this biomedical model, as we eat, food is broken down into glucose; this glucose makes its way into our cells as sources of energy. In order for the glucose to enter cells, insulin is necessary. Insulin is described by biomedical providers as the key that opens the pathway allowing glucose to enter the cell. For someone with diabetes, then, their insulin is not working the way that the biomedical model expects it should—it is not opening that cell, or the individual is not producing enough insulin. In these descriptions, we can see that there is an expectation for how the body should function and that with diabetes the body is not doing what is expected of it. The result of this lack of proper functioning or reduced amount of insulin is hyperglycemia. This model frames the disease around the metaphor of the body as a machine or factory of machines, in which the piece responsible for insulin production or the cells that should be responsive to insulin are defective. This body-as-machine metaphor is common in biomedical models of the body today.[33]

While this biomedical definition strives to describe the physiological factors behind diabetes, it does not get at the experience of the disease for those living with it in the same way that Aretæus was able to in the first century CE. Since that time, a great separation has occurred in biomedicine, whereby patients and their experience of disease have been removed from definitions of disease and findings based in the biotechnological sciences have taken the place of the patients and their bodily experiences.

In recent decades biomedical technologies have increasingly affected the human body's experience. Rayna Rapp describes how ultrasound technology has altered the ways in which women experience pregnancy.[34] Today, the health of the fetus that was once only known through the mother's experiences can be viewed through the technology; ultrasound, as Rapp explains, gives doctors a window into the womb and shifts the experience of pregnancy from an individual mother's experience to a communal one. This shift in bodily health experience is also noted in the work of Margaret Lock and Annemarie Mol, where the severity of brain death and atherosclerosis is defined through expert interpretation of high-tech images.[35] In the case of atherosclerosis, the person's experience of their own body is shaped by these expert interpretations.[36] Medical technologies are increasingly making their way into individual homes, and this migration is especially true for diabetes management. In her study of blood glucose monitoring devices in the Netherlands, Annemarie Mol shows that through the increase in at-home glucose monitoring, the sensations of hyperglycemia in diabetes patients are no longer trustworthy, taking a back seat to the numbers that appear on the screen.[37] In chapter 6 I discuss how some research participants with diabetes explain that they do not always feel any symptoms of the disease and are reliant upon these blood glucose monitoring devices to tell them if their blood glucose levels are in the range their physicians would like them to be. Technologies, then, not only shift views of the body but can also challenge and alter one's lived bodily experiences.

Biomedical technologies, in addition to shaping the personal experiences of disease, shape medical classification systems. As a medical technology, insulin shifted the experience of those living with diabetes. People with diabetes now live for decades after diagnosis, an increased lifespan that has led to further refinements in the biomedical model of diabetes. In the mid-twentieth century biomedical researchers began to record related complications: renal disease, retinopathy, cardiovascular disease, and neuropathy. By the 1970s research studies were associating long-term hyperglycemia with the development of these complications.[38] During this post–insulin therapy period, diabetes not only grew to include the possible development of future complications but was also redefined by researchers to include multiple forms of the condition. Until the 1930s biomedicine recognized diabetes as a single disease. By the end of the 1950s, researchers had noted variation in amounts of extractable insulin in diabetic patients through postmortem autopsies that suggested differing degrees of diabetes severity. By the 1980s it was well recognized that there are multiple forms of diabetes, forms that are continuing to expand today.[39] Over the course of sixty years, then, diabetes transitioned through insulin therapy from a fatal disease to a set of diseases that share hyperglycemia as a defining feature and that can lead to complications if not kept under control.

The three most common forms of diabetes are type 2, type 1, and gestational diabetes. According to the biomedical model, type 2 diabetes occurs in individuals who are insulin resistant. Often in the early stages of type 2 diabetes, insulin is overproduced, and the individual builds up a resistance to the hormone. In the past, type 2 diabetes was often referred to as adult-onset diabetes, because people typically developed the disease in mid-to-late adulthood. Today more and more people are developing this form of diabetes at a younger age, and Indigenous Americans have the highest rate of adolescent and childhood type 2 diabetes cases in the United States.[40] Two less common types of diabetes are type 1 and gestational diabetes. According to the biomedical model, type 1 diabetes occurs in individuals whose immune system destroyed the insulin producing cells of the pancreas, and gestational diabetes occurs when pregnancy induces a state of insulin resistance. In gestational diabetes, once the woman has given birth, her blood glucose returns to normal levels; however, both the mother and the child are considered to be at a heightened risk for developing type 2 diabetes later in life. There are additional forms of diabetes that are brought on by disease and surgery that occur less frequently, and there are multiple divisions within type 2 and type 1 being defined and elaborated upon each year by national and international diabetes organizations.[41]

To summarize, biomedicine defines diabetes as a chronic condition characterized by elevated levels of blood glucose due to either insulin deficiency or insulin resistance, which can lead to complications if not controlled. What biomedicine is still striving to answer is what the ultimate causes of diabetes are—why do some people become insulin resistant? And why do others lose their insulin producing cells? Before discussing hypotheses for type 2 diabetes etiology, I describe the recent history of diabetes in America's Indigenous populations.

The Indigenous American Diabetes Epidemic

While there is clear evidence of diabetes in human populations throughout the past thirty-five hundred years, diabetes was rare in Indigenous American populations prior to the mid-twentieth century. The earliest recorded case of diabetes in a Native person is found in the medical notes of Doctor W. K. Callahan, who treated an Akimel O'odham woman for diabetes in 1902.[42] The next recorded case is found in diabetes specialist Elliot P. Joslin's 1940 article "The Universality of Diabetes," in which he describes how diabetes is found among members of an Arizona Navajo population, noting one diabetic Navajo male specifically.[43] Based upon military records, Kelly M. West finds no recorded cases of diabetes prior to 1939 among Natives living in Oklahoma.[44] Both West's study and Dennis Wiedman's more recent study of federal Indian agents' records from the mid-nineteenth century on three southwestern tribes describe finding no cases of diabetes in Native populations in the nineteenth century.[45] Based on their archival work, I surmise that diabetes was documented in earlier Native populations; at the same time, it was very rare (if present at all) prior to the late nineteenth century. In the 1950s diabetes did not factor into the top ten causes of death for Native Americans based on Indian Health Service records. During that time, the service's programs were aimed toward the treatment and prevention of communicable diseases, like tuberculosis. By the late 1990s, however, diabetes was the fourth leading cause of death for Native Americans, listed behind heart disease, cancer, and accidents.[46]

Today Native American populations have some of the highest rates of diabetes in the world.[47] Due to disturbances in lifestyles brought on by European expansion and colonization, the growing rates of diabetes in indigenous populations is a global trend.[48] For the Indigenous American population of the United States, the majority of diabetes research and known rates are based upon Indian Health Service studies conducted in reservation clinics. Though there is less data on the diagnosis rates of diabetes in urban settings, it is prevalent in urban Native populations where studies have been completed; 19.8 percent of those over the age of forty-five in Los Angeles and 21 percent of those over the age of fifty in Seattle have been diagnosed with the disease.[49] I found in my own study that no published rates of diabetes for Chicago's Native population exist, and the feasibility of accurately estimating rates in the city is complicated by the fact that Chicago Natives utilize a wide variety of health-care providers both in the city and on reservations. Through interviews I learned that community health workers in Chicago hold widely varying estimates—one nurse guessed that as few as 10 percent of the population had diabetes, while another estimated that it was nearly 80 percent.

As I have noted, rates of diabetes in Indigenous American populations have grown drastically over the past sixty years and are estimated by the CDC to be higher than the rates of diabetes in other ethnic populations.[50] However, while talking about diabetes in the community during an unrecorded interview, an employee of American Indian Health Service of Chicago posed a question to me—are rates of diabetes in Native peoples that much higher than the rates in other ethnic populations, or are the rates similar but only seen as higher in Native populations because of the higher level of reports on Native health statuses through the Indian Health Service? This individual had stated earlier in our conversation that diabetes is one of the leading causes of death in Natives, but he further believed cases of diabetes in other ethnic populations are equally high. This man's question raises an important point—Indigenous American bodies have been, as Michel Foucault might say, under surveillance since the eighteenth century.[51] Is it the case that rates of diabetes are similar to other populations, but appear higher in Native populations because of this surveillance? I do not have an answer to this question, but it deserves some serious consideration.

Ethnographers have documented how published health and disease data are shaped by local history, culture, and politics. In the United States, Roy Grinker asks if there are really more cases of autism spectrum disorder in recent years, or if it is the case that the number of cases remains unchanged but the disorder itself is more visible through the increased number of services available.[52] Ian Whitmarsh's study of asthma in Barbados illustrates the role society and history play in the diagnosis of a chronic condition. The West Indian island of Barbados has a high occurrence of asthma, with up to 20 percent of its population being affected by the disease. Barbados has a national contract with a biomedical research team from the United States; because of this, Whitmarsh questions whether there are really comparatively more cases of asthma in Barbados as the statistics suggest, or if these numbers are the result of greater awareness due to this research relationship.[53] Steve Ferzacca's ethnography on health in modern Indonesia illustrates how Suharto's New Order regime strove to demonstrate the modernity and development of Indonesia by citing increasing national rates of chronic conditions like heart disease, hypertension, and diabetes. At the same time, however, doctors in the Javanese city where Ferzacca worked describe that 50 percent of the cases they regularly encountered were cases of infectious diseases like dengue fever, malaria, and tuberculosis.[54] Based on the findings of Ferzacca, Whitmarsh, and Grinker, the question posed by the staff member at American Indian Health Service of Chicago on the difference in rates of diabetes by ethnicity deserves attention and sincere consideration that are outside the scope of this book.

Explaining the Recent Rise

In populations that had comparatively low rates of diabetes sixty years ago, why has the disease become an epidemic over the course of a few decades? In the remainder of this chapter, I engage with literature from the biological sciences that has aimed to answer this question and suggest how social science perspectives contribute to these discussions. I focus on the two mainstream biomedical explanations for diabetes development—genetic and phenotypic features and environmental factors—and argue that scientists investigating the cause of the recent diabetes epidemic in Native populations must take colonial history and policies into account.

Thrifty Genotypes and Phenotypes

In 1962 geneticist James Neel postulated the existence of a thrifty genotype that helped earlier humans to survive a turbulent history by allowing for the storage of excess fat during periods of feast to live off of in times of famine. While this genotype was beneficial in the past, it has become detrimental in an era of constant food supply.[55] Neel did not initially link his thrifty genotype hypothesis to Native American populations, but the researchers behind a longitudinal study of diabetes among the Akimel O'odham believed that the concept adequately explained the recent epidemic rise in the number of diabetes cases among Native American groups.[56] Later in his career Neel agreed with these researchers, applying his hypothesis to the Indigenous populations of North and South America.[57]

More than three decades after Neel's first publication of the hypothesis, biological anthropologists John Allen and Susan Cheer describe it as ethnocentric, arguing that the model describes the thrifty genotype as a derived trait rather than an ancestral one, meaning that Neel hypothesized that earlier humans shared a non-thrifty genotype and later humans developed a thrifty genotype.[58] Allen and Cheer argue that it was more likely that all human ancestors shared the thrifty genotype as a primitive trait and that the nonthrifty genotype later developed in contexts with more reliable food supplies. There have been further critiques of Neel from the biological sciences, the most significant of which is the lack of genetic evidence to support his hypothesis.[59] Still, this lack of evidence does not mean that there is no genetic basis for type 2 diabetes, as genetic research has identified many genes related to the condition.[60]

Thirty years after Neel's first publication on the thrifty genotype hypothesis, biochemist C. Nicholas Hales and physician epidemiologist David Barker posited that rather than a thrifty genotype, a thrifty phenotype was a more feasible model for understanding diabetes etiology. According to this hypothesis, humans are predisposed to diabetes not by genes but by development in early stages of life. Hales and Barker contend, "Poor nutrition of the fetus and infant leads to permanent changes of the structure and function of certain organs and tissues . . . we suggest that poor early development of islets of Langerhans and β cells is a major factor in the etiology of Type 2 diabetes."[61] The thrifty phenotype hypothesis argues that a rapid shift from low birth weight and poor fetal nutrition to overnutrition in early life may lead to glucose intolerance later in life. They further note that this hypothesis does not remove genes entirely from the diabetes etiology picture, finding that the genes involved in fetal development may play a significant role in diabetes development. While Neel's thrifty genotype hypothesis has lost popular support in the past few decades, Hale and Barker's thrifty phenotype alternative is more widely accepted in the biomedical research community.[62]

Both hypotheses consider biological makeup as one piece in the puzzle of diabetes etiology. For many researchers, diabetes is a biocultural condition, a disease to which one is predisposed by biological factors and that is then triggered by a cultural environment.[63]

Environment and Life Conditions

Biomedical providers interviewed for this study held varied views of what causes diabetes. Some argued for both a genetic and environmental component, while others focused entirely on environment—

citing diet, obesity, work life, low physical activity, poverty, food deserts, lack of education, stress, and intergenerational trauma. Many biological studies argue that a decrease in physical activity plays a significant role in the development of diabetes, and that diets high in fat and refined carbohydrates are behind the epidemic in Native populations.[64] In a comparative study of diabetes rates in two related Native populations living on different sides of the United States-Mexico border, Leslie Schulz found that among the Akimel O'odham living a more "traditional lifestyle" in Mexico, eating foods higher in fiber and being more physically active prevented the emergence of diabetes in that population.[65] Schulz here employs the term "lifestyle," which is commonly used in literature theorizing the cause for diabetes development. This use of the term particularly in relation to the Indigenous American diabetes epidemic is problematic. Susan Reynolds Whyte challenges its use when speaking of noncommunicable chronic diseases. She argues that the use of the term glosses over political and social situations, in which many of these so-called lifestyle factors are not the result of choice but are due to circumstances outside the control of individuals developing noncommunicable chronic conditions. Whyte proposes using the term "life conditions" instead of "lifestyle."[66]

I take a biocultural approach to understanding the recent rise of diabetes in the Indigenous populations of the Americas. Human history, politics, and society play a role in shaping human biology and health. For Indigenous American populations, colonial history and policies have played a significant role in shaping their contemporary health. Diseases and epidemics of disease are situated within local political, social histories. Anthropologists Mariana K. Leal Ferreira, Gretchen Chesley Lang, and Nancy Scheper-Hughes argue that biological studies and theorizations, like the thrifty genotype hypothesis, depoliticize the colonial histories of forced movement that led to the disease; as these anthropologists argue, the shift in Indigenous American diabetes cases is largely related to life changes imposed upon Indigenous peoples by Western colonial forces.[67] The critique Scheper-Hughes and Ferreria and

Lang level at these biological scientists is supported by researchers studying the effect of colonialism on the bodies of the Indigenous peoples of the Americas.

Indeed, forced changes in life conditions led to the diabetes epidemic among Native Americans today. According to Winnebago nurse Lorelei de Cora, the United States federal government holds a large portion of the responsibility for this phenomenon; she points out that Indigenous peoples became dependent upon federally allocated food supplies due to restrictions on land area—supplies that consisted of foods lacking nutritional value and containing high levels of fat and simple carbohydrates.[68] Yvonne Jackson describes the change in the general diet of Indigenous peoples since colonization and forced relocation: "The diets today are high in refined carbohydrates, fat, and sodium, and are low in meats, eggs, cheese, milk, vegetables, and fruits. Many dishes are combinations of meat and starch, and many foods are fried."[69] In addition to changes in diet, de Cora describes how the land restriction greatly decreased the amount of physical activity that individuals performed on a daily basis.[70] According to Betty Geishirt Cantrell, the Sioux diet based on the local agriculture and strenuous labor was replaced during the period of relocation to reservations with a diet high in white flour, sugar, and lard.[71] James Justice adds to de Cora's, Jackson's, and Geishirt Cantrell's arguments by indicating that these changes in diet were largely associated with socioeconomic standing; the movement to reservations forced Natives into a socioeconomic position where they became dependent on the federal government for food provisions.[72]

While rates of diabetes climbed in reservation spaces in the decades following World War II, they simultaneously grew in city spaces. Many Native migrants faced financial hardship after moving to the city, and while some returned to the reservation, others continued to reside in the city and make their way with the support of other Natives and urban Native organizations. Rebecca, a fifty-three-year-old Odawa/Omaha woman and second-generation urban Native, described how her parents at one time lived in a one-bedroom apartment with eleven other adults and Rebecca as an infant. Growing up, however, Rebecca did not realize that her family struggled financially:

REBECCA: I never knew we were poor. One time I asked my mom, and this was like ten years ago, mom you used to make really good potato soup. I said how come you don't make that anymore, and she said because we were poor. We were poor? We were poor, but we always had food from the garden and I remember [my father would] buy a half a beef at a time. We never went without anything. I just didn't realize.

Not all families had the opportunity to grow a garden while living in the Chicago region, as Rebecca's family did. Oral history interviewees describe that their families faced greater difficulty in eating healthier meals after relocating to the city than they did on the reservation. In part, this was because their families had more space for growing gardens on their home reservation than they did in the city. Arlene, a sixty-three-year-old Ojibwe/Odawa woman described:

ARLENE: We didn't have much money at the time . . . we didn't have much money at the time so we lived in the car . . . moving here was hard at the beginning for my mom . . . No one would eat it nowadays, but we used to eat cornmeal mush. There was a lot of it then. It was cheap, so my mom made us that.

Paul Farmer has championed the application of Johan Galtung's concept of structural violence to understand the occurrence of health inequities. In his 1969 paper on peace studies, Galtung defines structural violence as violence that is committed by no direct actor.[73] Farmer extends Galtung's conceptualization in his work by investigating the ways in which societal structures—like those of race, gender, class, and religion—inflict violence by shaping health and access to health care for communities around the globe.[74] For America's Indigenous peoples, it is certainly the history of colonial policies and violence shaping contemporary Native health, as well as societal structures. I argue that diabetes in Native American peoples is the embodiment of the structural violence brought on by colonialism in the centuries following European-American contact with the Indigenous populations of North America.

The scholarship on the diabetes epidemic from both cultural and biological standpoints is significant, but is greatly lacking in two important areas. First, most biological studies on the factors behind diabetes in Native American populations tends to focus on the individual bodies—on their genotypes, phenotypes, individual activity level, and diet. What these studies do not consider is the role of history in shaping these bodies and the role of colonialism behind the epidemic. Social scientists and Native scholars have brought to light the central role colonialism has played in the recent diabetes epidemic in Native populations, and its importance to diabetes research. As I will show in the following chapter, it affects the ways in which people think about diabetes and subsequently treat it. Second, the majority of the research has focused on reservation populations. While rates of diabetes climbed in reservation areas, they also grew in cities, where the majority of Indigenous Americans live today, an experience I delve into in the next chapter.

4

Diabetes in Native Chicago

The receptionist's authoritative voice traveled through the ceiling and into the background of our conversation, as Idella and I spoke in a basement office at the American Indian Center. We had tried to escape the heat of the July afternoon by moving to the basement, but there was little relief to be found in the humid space. Idella is a thirty-five-year-old Potawatomi/Puerto Rican woman. She was diagnosed with type 2 diabetes just one month prior to our interview. Wearing an oversized navy-blue Chicago Cubs T-shirt with black ankle-length leggings, Idella rested her arms on the table between us as she described the effect diabetes has had on her family. She listed family members living with the disease, naming her grandmother, mother, aunts, and uncles. Later in our conversation Idella related her growing concern for her teenage daughter, who was beginning to display dark patches of skin on the back of her neck—a sign many mothers in the community regard as an early symptom of diabetes in children.[1] We spoke about her care routine and the adjustments she has made since her own diagnosis. In response to one of the last questions— what she wants to see for her own and the community's future— Idella returned to her concern over the high rates of diabetes in her family and in the community:

IDELLA: Honestly, like all the people that I know that are Native American and that are family, everybody has it. It's just something, I don't know if it's in our blood, from our generations, but everybody that I know familywise or friends that are Native American all have diabetes . . . for us it's like in our blood I think and it's passed down from generation to generation, 'cause you know my mom passed it down to me and I kind of passed it down to my older daughter and now I'm scared, because, if she don't lose the weight, she's going to be with diabetes.

While there are no published statistics on rates of diabetes in Chicago's Native population, accounts like Idella's attest to the high prevalence of diabetes in the community today.

Diabetes has been in Chicago's Native community since the beginning of the Urban Indian Relocation Program in the 1950s, becoming a pressing health concern by the 1980s. Ada Powers, a participant in the 1980s Chicago American Indian Oral History Pilot Project, described in a 1983 interview how nearly all Chicago Natives are affected by diabetes: "To me it seems like all the Indians are crippled or diabetics. I'm one of them. If it's just the Indian himself or their diets or what, but all those old Indians you talk to, they're diabetic . . . No matter who you talk to, they got diabetes."[2] While Idella's statement mirrors that of Ada Powers from nearly thirty years earlier, Idella also speaks to the contemporary spread of diabetes among the younger generations. Children as young as eleven years old are being diagnosed as prediabetic, making the condition a significant health concern for Chicago Natives of all ages.

My aim in this chapter is to build upon the broader history described in the preceding one by introducing diabetes in Native Chicago. I show that its prevalence shapes local beliefs, care and prevention practices, and understandings of the condition. I first describe how community members learn about diabetes in childhood. I then show that, in conjunction with public health media, the prevalence of the disease fosters the idea of heightened risk of diabetes in Native populations and that this labeling can foster fatalistic views about the condition's development. In the third section I describe the moralization of diabetes care practices and management. Finally, I examine a local taxonomy of diabetes severity, demonstrating that the classification of diabetes forms is situated within local experiences with the disease.

Developing an Awareness of Diabetes in Childhood

In July 2009 wellness staff at the American Indian Center chose diabetes as their monthly health topic. Every month, members of the wellness staff would provide information on a specific health topic via lectures, handouts, and demonstrations to senior lunch attendees, with the aim of educating seniors about common health concerns in the community. Topics in the past included cancer, heart disease, and men's and women's health. When Wendy presented on diet and diabetes, she did so to more than fifty people in attendance at the elder lunch. During her presentation she asked members of the audience—a mix of both seniors and youth and of Natives and non-Natives—to raise their hands if they had an immediate family member with diabetes. Nearly every person in Tribal Hall that day raised a hand.

This scene illustrates the situation described by Idella and Ada Powers. There is a high rate of diabetes in Chicago's Native community, and not only are adults aware of this prevalence but so too are the children attending the summer youth program. In contrast to the non-Native medical providers I spoke with, Native medical providers, diabetics, and lay caregivers were often conscious of what diabetes was from childhood. Whereas non-Natives first learned of the disease in school, Native participants often recalled seeing a relative inject themselves with insulin, test their blood glucose levels, limit the foods they eat, and/or contend with diabetes complications, which can include the loss of limbs and eyesight.

For Native youth in Chicago, diabetes is ever present in their lifeworld, which stands in stark contrast to that of Native peoples seventy years ago, when diabetes was rare. Alfred Schutz describes the lifeworld as the intersubjective world of everyday life of an individual, which puts people, phenomena, objects, concepts, stories, history, et cetera within an individual's reach.[3] The constitution of the "world of daily life" is not chosen or developed by the individual but is created through their continuous interactions in the world.[4] Kenneth George builds upon Schutz when he describes a lifeworld as "the ongoing circumstances in which we find ourselves, culturally, politically, historically, and experientially. Each of us is thrown, with others, into a lifeworld through which we must find our way, refashioning its horizons as imaginatively and as pragmatically as we can."[5] Lifeworlds are intersubjective, always in motion, partial, and, at times, inconsistent.[6] In contemporary Native Chicago, diabetes often makes its way into the lifeworlds of individuals early in life. In the city, Natives learn about diabetes through relationships of care within their families, often at a comparatively young age when contrasted with non-Natives.

Adults in the community recall their first awareness of diabetes through witnessing either the care or the complications of the disease in their family. Diane remembered growing up around diabetes:

DIANE: My aunt had diabetes, and that was my mom's best friend, my dad's sister. I remember she always used to give herself insulin shots and so we al-, I mean she'd kind of, we knew she had diabetes, I mean she had to take insulin shots. We knew that's all we seen, that's all we knew about it when I was little . . . I learned more about it as I got older, like I'd ask questions. [twenty-seven-year-old Arikara/Omaha/Odawa woman]

Diane's description of observing her aunt take shots mirrors the experience of others who also sought further information as they grew older. Diabetes was witnessed not only in households but also in the community. Those who did not have family members with the disease recollect first learning of the condition through friends and community members. Debbie recalls having a young friend with diabetes:

DEBBIE: A young man, a Native man many years ago, his name was Alan . . . he had it. And that's how I really knew what the heck was going on because then I found out it was really bad because he started losing his limbs, he went blind, and he started . . . that's the first time I ever knew about it and it was twenty something years ago. [forty-seven-year-old Ho-Chunk woman with diabetic family members]

For members of Chicago's Native community, learning about diabetes in childhood shapes the ways in which they understand, and in some cases care for, diabetes later in life. This care work shapes how people think about diabetes, and for many members of Chicago's Native community, then, the process of learning about diabetes is embedded in relationships of caring for kin. This process of learning is distinctly different from many that of the biomedically trained caregivers seen by diabetes patients in the community, who often first learn about this disease through studying its pathologies in school, and later building upon this knowledge through the practice of applying their medical knowledge to patient care. Helena, a sixty-eight-year-old Apache woman living with diabetes, explained that she first learned of the disease and of disease care through helping others in her youth and that this trained and prepared her for caring for diabetes later in life:

HELENA: You get more the severeness of the diabetes in one respect [from doctors]. Family you get the real stuff. You get what you can have, what it's about [from doctors], but with family you get what it is. There's that difference, another interpretation.

Throughout her life, Helena has learned about diabetes from multiple sources—from popular media, from biomedical encounters, from pamphlets and informational brochures, from friends, and from family. As she explained, her family's experiences with diabetes and its care inform and shape her care practices.

Diabetes Risk and Fatalistic Views

Pine-scented floor cleaner permeated the air on a warm June 2009 morning as staff and community members of Chicago's American

Indian Center gathered in Tribal Hall for the biweekly elder lunch. The table for health screenings stood at the back of this expansive space and was ready for business, with medical supplies arranged neatly for use. I sat at this table with Violet, a retired registered nurse who volunteers for the center's wellness department, providing health screenings for any member or visitor interested in having their blood pressure and/or blood glucose measured. Just before lunch began, a middle-aged Native woman took the seat to Violet's left. After checking her blood pressure, Violet asked if she would like to have her blood glucose measured. The woman responded in the negative, stating "I don't have diabetes, thank god." After a brief pause the woman finished her statement with a decisive "yet." I jotted down the woman's words and found myself pondering the meaning behind this "yet" upon my return home that evening. Does she believe that it is inevitable that she will develop the disease? And what has led to such an outlook?

In the years that followed that lunch, I continued to hear similar statements from people of all ages. Chris, a forty-five-year-old Potawatomi/Puerto Rican man, described how all but one of his siblings had developed diabetes by their early forties, and that it was only a matter of time before that last sibling developed it. James, an employee at the American Indian Center in his late twenties, would occasionally stop by the health screening table to test his blood glucose levels. James frequently had low readings—indicating hypoglycemia, the reverse of the characteristic trait of diabetes, hyperglycemia. After several weeks of his stopping by the health screening table, I asked him why he frequently checked his blood glucose and if he had diabetes. Without hesitation, James replied that he did not have diabetes but was sure that he would have it by the age of thirty-five; he then left the table in search of some juice to correct his low blood glucose level. The sentiments expressed by James, Chris, and the woman at the health screening table demonstrate the widespread belief in a high diabetes risk in the community.

This conception of risk is not only due to the ubiquity of diabetes: it is further heightened and shaped by public health campaigns.

In the first few years of this study, when the American Indian Center employed a wellness department with nurses and dieticians, there were multiple informational sheets, pamphlets, and posters around the common areas of the center for community members to take home with them. Pamphlets like these factor greatly into the knowledge base of community members, who describe family experience, biomedical encounters, and literature as being among their top resources for diabetes knowledge.

Most of the health-related media I noted at the center focused on the topics of heart disease and diabetes. The latter offered information on controlling and preventing the disease. Pamphlets from the American Diabetes Association and the National Diabetes Education Program offered hope for prevention, with statements like: "You can prevent and control diabetes"; "But you can stay healthy and have fun by keeping active"; and "We must take charge of diabetes—for future generations." At the same time, in these same pamphlets and posters the messages of hope and support were preceded by descriptions of Natives as being at high risk for diabetes, for example, "Type 2 diabetes is more common than ever in young American Indians and Native Alaskans," and "Diabetes is a growing problem for Native Americans. Many Native Americans have Type II diabetes." Informational pamphlets provide risk factors for readers to reflect upon and calculate individual risk, describing people who have diabetic family members, who are overweight, and who are over the age of thirty as being particularly vulnerable.

In the world of modern epidemiology, everyone is at risk.[7] Nikolas Rose explains that, in the last decades of the twentieth century, the responsibility has shifted to the individual to care for and manage risk in the growing world of chronic disease.[8] Indigenous Americans have been defined and labeled as a group at risk of developing diabetes, and this labeling has had the lasting effect of altering Native perspectives of the world. In Puneet Chawla Sahota's study on a southwestern reservation, she found that in a community where James Neel's thrifty genotype hypothesis in relation to Native diabetes development is commonly cited as a cause for the epidemic, 22 percent of the fifty-three people she interviewed held fatalistic views about diabetes development.[9] The thrifty genotype hypothesis was not cited by Chicago Natives in their explanations for diabetes. I argue here, however, that pamphlets with covers asking readers: "Diabetes and American Indians: Are You at Risk?" similarly contribute to local conceptions of diabetes risk and fatalistic views.

As is evident in the statements from James, Chris, and the woman at the health screening table, fatalistic views of diabetes development are common in Native Chicago. Community members' fatalistic views of the disease are shaped by the ubiquity of diabetes and by public health media. Yet, while holding a fatalistic view is often linked to inaction, this is not the case for resigned views about diabetes development in Native Chicago.

In a discussion of East Asian fatalistic beliefs, Arthur Niehoff defines fatalism as the view that an event is fated to happen and that nothing can be done to alter or prevent it.[10] Similarly, in *Tuhami*, an ethnographic portrait of a Moroccan man, Vincent Crapanzano describes his close informant Tuhami's fatalistic view of life.[11] Tuhami believed that his destiny in love was entirely left up to Allah and the saints. This view frustrated Crapanzano, who wanted to see this close informant married. Crapanzano describes his realization of Tuhami's passive submission to this belief in fated futures, predetermined and arranged by higher powers, as a turning point in his fieldwork toward a more therapeutic relationship with this informant.

In the case of Tuhami, a fatalistic view resulted in a passive life stance. But such an outcome is not predetermined. In Chicago's Native community, I found a mix of responses to fatalistic conceptions of diabetes. There are people who believe they will develop diabetes and do not take action to change their lives to prevent it. There are also people who believe they will develop the disease but adjust their lifestyle by eating what they consider healthier foods and increasing physical activity to prolong the time between the healthy present and the condition's onset. And though fatalistic views are widespread, there are some who make life adjustments with the expectation that they can and will prevent the development of diabetes altogether. Virginia, a thirty-one-year-old Navajo woman with a family history of diabetes, told me she aims to avoid diabetes by making a series of changes in her life. These include being physically active on a regular basis, eating whole grain foods, cooking with olive oil, and even making frybread with whole wheat flour in place of white. So, while fatalistic views about the disease are prevalent in Native Chicago, many people are actively engaging in lifestyle activities meant to either prevent the disease entirely or to extend the time before its development.

Stigma and Moralizing Discourse of Care

The response to any condition or disease is situated within time and space. This fact is explored in Ruth Benedict's 1934 essay on the "Anthropology of the Abnormal," where she describes the role played by cultural models of understanding in determining whether a mental state or a behavioral pattern is normal or is not—an argument highlighting the Boasian notion of cultural relativism in the field of cultural anthropology.[12] As Benedict demonstrates, a person experiencing seizures and trance may be defined as severely ill in one society, while taking on the role of a shaman in another. The experience and response to human states of health and illness are dependent upon location and time. In the case of diabetes, its development is increasingly becoming stigmatized in different regions of the world. People view diabetes as a preventable disease and the blame is often placed on individual life choices, like diet, which are often outside the control of those being blamed.[13] Yet, in the context of Native Chicago, the development of diabetes does not hold the same social stigma. Forty-one-year-old Oneida citizen and Chicago community health worker Dacia explained:

DACIA: Diabetes has some social stigmas outside of Native community, I think. Type 2 diabetes, definitely, there's social stigmas. In the Native communities, not so much.

While there is no stigma associated with developing the disease in the community, there is a heightened level of criticism for those who are viewed as not taking care of the disease once they have it. This criticism is found in local discourse that moralizes the behaviors of people known to be living with diabetes, focusing in particular on the consumption choices that known diabetics make. Agnes, who has had diabetes since the 1970s, offered a commentary on how one of her close friends cares for the disease:

AGNES: My friend Sarah was diabetic. She was a diabetic too. But we used to have fun. I would go all the way to Flint, Michigan, to visit her from here on weekends. She was so nice. But diabetes is nothing to play with. Some people think just because they're taking pills or taking shots they can eat anything, which they shouldn't. I tell myself that. Just because you're taking pills doesn't mean you can eat anything. Because it's still in your blood. Your, your blood sugar goes up three . . . , in the three hundreds, not mine, these are other people now. They take their blood sugar and it's, sometimes it's four hundred. That one, the one I'm talking about, she's in South Dakota right now. She comes around here, when she comes back, she'll come around again. Hers is real bad.

MEG: And is it because she just eats what she wants?

AGNES: Eats what she wants.

MEG: Yeah.

AGNES: Oh and she always has a bottle of soft drinks, one of the quarts.

MEG: But not diet, regular?

AGNES: No not diet, regular. She has candy, cookies, and she eats anything. [eighty-two-year-old Odawa woman]

Here, Agnes was critical both of her friend's consumption of foods that diabetics are typically forewarned against eating in excess and of her elevated blood glucose levels. With several decades of experience managing her own case of diabetes, Agnes described Sarah's actions as a failure to manage the disease properly. This was the most common critique people used when speaking of those who do not take care of diabetes—they are consuming foods that the interviewee does not think they should. The practice of moralizing about food consumption in the United States has been described in other contexts, particularly in those pertaining to women's bodies.[14] In Chicago, many community members—both those living with and not living with diabetes—describe situations where they comment on or "nag" those with diabetes whom they see eating foods they believe are bad for them.

The expectation in the community is that people learn how to care for the disease and follow the steps to do so. Overhearing a conversation I was having with a former American Indian Center employee about my plans to attend a training session offered by Rush University Medical Center to learn about the Stanford University course "Take Charge of Your Diabetes," which aims to provide general diabetes information while promoting individual care, Chris, who was passing through the center's kitchen, stopped to join in our discussion. Chris offered his opinion, stating that people who have diabetes should already know everything about how to treat and care for it, implying the course would not be of need in the community. Moralizing discourse about diabetes care is found in other contexts, in which diabetes patients describe themselves as not fulfilling their patient duties by complying with doctor's orders.[15] In Native Chicago, not only are diabetes patients and medical providers discussing diabetes care and compliance in moralizing terms, but so too are nondiabetic community members when speaking about their friends and family members' care practices. In addition to this set of management expectations for those who have it, there is a local model for understanding levels of diabetes severity.

A Local Model of Categorizing Diabetes

I spoke with Charles, an active member of the center, on a great number of occasions about diabetes, diabetes prevention, and healthy eating. Charles is a proponent of eating the diet of one's ancestors, and in his case as a thirty-one-year-old Sioux man, he had been experimenting with a low-carbohydrate and high-lean-protein diet. In a formal interview, Charles began to describe his role in his partner's diabetes care when he brought up a term for diabetes with which I was unfamiliar:

> CHARLES: Well I know Aria, the mother of my son, she's already diabetic, type 2 diabetes, but she's already on, on the path to being full-blown diabetic. She's having to take insulin now . . .
>
> MEG: Can I ask what you mean by full-blown diabetic?
>
> CHARLES: I would say somebody that has to take, where their pancreas is ready to shut down. I don't know if that's how it would be defined or what. I mean I'm not even sure. The, I feel like the term diabetes is very ambiguous and it, there should be more defined terminology besides type 1 diabetes, type 2 diabetes, and whatever else . . . The way I view it is that there is a whole spectrum of sensitivity towards these foods. Some people are more sensitive than others obviously. Some people are more sensitive to other things as well.

Charles's description of diabetes as being organized less by distinct types and more along a spectrum represents one aspect of the local classification system of diabetes in Native Chicago. Based on descriptions from individuals living with diabetes and individuals who have the condition in their family, I describe the local classification system, which looks at the disease as falling along a spectrum, moving from mild cases to more severe. In the previous chapter I described how the biomedical diabetes classification system has mushroomed over the past century since the development of insulin therapy for diabetes patients—distinguishing manifestations of diabetes by distinctive types. Local diabetes classification differs from those of published biomedical materials, in that it is organized by care needs and the effect diabetes has on life.

Local categories of diabetes are shaped by individual lifeworlds, that is, what people observe in the community, and these categories, in turn, shape action. This local diabetes classification system resonates with theorizations on human knowledge and cognition. Organization of human thought is shaped by local environments; for instance, Harold Conklin explains that color perceptions are influenced by one's context, finding that the Hanunoo have multiple levels of color classifications that are shaped by their engagements with the local environment.[16] In a similar vein Michelle Rosaldo describes that the Illongot created a taxonomic system to define their local plant life. While she found that there is some looseness with the terms used in this system to categorize orchid plants, there was a much more rigid set of organization for distinguishing one type of pea plant from another, and this is because some of the pea species in the area where Illongot live are fatal if consumed.[17] In her work several decades later, Anna Tsing demonstrates that nature knowledge is produced through specific forms of engagement with the surrounding world. As she argues, there is no pure or distinct natural environment; human knowledge of natural landscapes develops through practices of engagement and experience within it. In her ethnography, Tsing illustrates that humans approach and engage with nature in multiple ways. In the Meratus landscapes, for example, capitalist planners see a strict boundary between a forest and a field.[18] Those living in the Meratus landscapes, however, see multiple levels between the planners' bounded entities through their everyday engagement with their surroundings; women and children study and utilize the plant life growing in the "wild" swiddens. In their study of the International Classification of Diseases, Geoffrey Bowker and Susan Leigh Star build upon these descriptions of human cognitive organization to show that the processes of defining classifications can be invisible.[19]

While classifications are based upon engagement, human action is in turn organized by classification systems. In his study of Nuer and Tikopea classification systems for twins, animals, birds, and vegetables, Raymond Firth explains that such systems influence human action and relationships with objects in their environment.[20] Ian Hacking demonstrates that the things that people do are intimately tied to the descriptive categories of society; the categories that a society has to describe ways of being, in effect, make up people. Hacking argues that these categories of being have their own history of coming into creation that is tightly bound to society, politics, and environment. While there are material and natural limitations to the emergence of categories, they come to gain meaning through the processes of naming.[21] Human classification systems, then, are built upon human engagement with their local environs, and these classification systems in turn play a role in shaping human behavior.

Of particular relevance to the present study, classifications shape human understandings of disease and human health care practices. Charles Frake describes the diagnosis of an ailment among the Subanun as a pivotal step in the medical process; once the diagnosis is made, treatment can be determined and implemented.[22] In a study of health care in an institutionalized medical setting, Linda Hunt and Nedal Arar describe how medical providers and patients have differing understandings of disease. As they explain, while doctors acquire knowledge of the chronic condition experience through tests, relying upon technology, patients gain knowledge through constantly living with the disease.[23] In their study of medical classifications of health and disease, Bowker and Star note that there is not a great divide between folk and scientific classifications of disease, and further, that there is some fluidity and movement between the two.[24] Based on this literature, it should come as no surprise that local understandings of diabetes are informed by and differ from biomedical understandings of the condition. Here, I describe how the emic, or insider, classification of diabetes forms differs from etic, or outsider, biomedical classifications (see tables 1 and 2).

The two most prominent differences between the models are, first, that the emic model is focused on distinguishing different forms of diabetes that would all fit within what are designated as

Table 1. Emic classifications

Referred to as	Includes
Borderline	At high risk of developing diabetes, but not diagnosed with diabetes. No pharmaceutical intervention necessary. Some people attempt to stop the disease progression.
Mild or not bad	Diagnosed with diabetes. Treated with diet and/or exercise alone.
Diabetes	Diagnosed with diabetes. Treated with prescribed oral medications, along with diet and/or exercise.
Full-blown or bad	Diagnosed with diabetes. Treated with insulin injections, along with prescribed oral medication, diet, and/or exercise.
Severe	Diagnosed with diabetes. Treated with insulin, prescribed oral medications, diet, and/or exercise. Developed diabetes complications (e.g., toe or limb amputated, lost eyesight, or on dialysis due to kidney failure).

Table 2. Etic classifications

Referred to as	Includes
Borderline or prediabetes	Slightly elevated glucose levels, but not high enough to be classified as diabetes (to be diagnosed with diabetes, one must have an $A_1C \geq 6.5$ or a fasting plasma glucose ≥ 126). Physicians recommend weight loss, exercise, and diet to prevent the transition of a borderline case into type 2 diabetes. In some circumstances, oral medications are prescribed, though this practice is controversial in the United States.
Type 2	Insulin resistant. Treatment is determined based on individual needs; can include diet, exercise, oral medications, and/or insulin injections.
Type 1	Insulin levels are low or absent. Requires insulin injections for survival. Treatment additionally includes diet and exercise, and can include oral medications in later life.

type 2 and borderline diabetes in the etic model. Second, this emic classification is organized around treatment needs—the more invasive the treatment, the more severe the case of diabetes—while the etic system is organized around the body's insulin production and reception capabilities in addition to treatment needs. In this section I show that the emic model is based upon local engagements with diabetes experience and care in the community and that this classification system is both developed and maintained through local discourse about diabetes care and experiences.

In table 1, borderline diabetes is defined as a case of diabetes not requiring medical intervention. Ruby, a sixty-four-year-old Menominee woman with diabetes, explained why the biomedical diagnosis of diabetes as borderline yet requiring medical intervention does not make sense:

> RUBY: Well they say it was borderline diabetes, but I take a pill . . .
> But I figure once borderline, you are or you're not. If you're taking
> the pill you are, you know. That's how I figure . . . why am I taking
> a pill if I'm borderline?

As seen in table 2, pharmaceutical intervention for borderline cases of diabetes is controversial in the biomedical world, but it does happen. Meta Kreiner and Linda Hunt describe that this conflation of risk with disease is increasingly common in biomedical contexts, in which physicians turn to aggressive treatment rather than preventative measures.[25] In *Drugs for Life*, Joseph Dumit fleshes out the ways in which the standards for disease cutoffs are constantly being scaled back to increase the pharmaceutical consumer population, thereby increasing drug sales in the United States.[26] In Chicago's Native community, borderline diabetes is described as being at high risk, but not having diabetes. Prescribed medication indicates a real shift from not having diabetes to having it. Individual responses to having borderline diabetes vary. After her eleven-year-old daughter was diagnosed as being on the border line of diabetes, Tiffany changed the child's diet to both help her lose weight and prevent her from developing the disease. In contrast, Joan was diagnosed with borderline diabetes, and while she changed her eating habits for a brief period of time, she explains that she eventually returned to her old habits of having a candy bar now and then. A year after her borderline diagnosis, Joan was diagnosed with diabetes, and attributes this shift in her health status to her eating habits over that year.

In the emic classification system, a mild case of diabetes is one in which a person does not have to take any medication, orally or via injections, and relies instead upon diet and other lifestyle changes. Carmen, a sixty-nine-year-old Oneida woman who has been living with diabetes for fifteen years, explained how if you work early on at diabetes care through lifestyle changes, it is not as severe a case:

> CARMEN: If you follow good eating habits, you know actually if you're not real, real bad in diabetics, you can, well you can't get rid of it, but you can get it where you don't have to take medication.

Now more than thirty years since her diagnosis, Tammy described that earlier in her life with diabetes, she was able to manage the disease through diet alone. During this time, the condition was so completely under control that she for a time forgot that she had diabetes. It was only when she was prescribed steroids for an unrelated health concern that her memory of having diabetes was roused. Tammy had not informed the prescribing doctor that she had diabetes. Steroids increase blood glucose levels; when Tammy took them, her blood glucose levels rose so considerably that she was hospitalized for a few days.

Moving from mild cases, diabetes gets classified as progressively worse in relation to increasingly invasive treatment. A case requiring oral medication is not labeled with a distinctive classification name, and the need for insulin is described as related to "full-blown" or "bad" cases of diabetes. Phillip, a fifty-two-year-old Micmac man with diabetes, explained that his wife, who takes insulin, has a case of what he terms "full-blown" diabetes:

> PHILLIP: And plus, you become a full, full, full-blown diabetics at any moment. That happened to my wife also, you know, so now

she got to get up every morning and shot in her stomach with a needle you know, and I'm trying to avoid that myself, you know.

From full-blown, cases become more severe when someone has a physical limitation brought on by the disease. Virginia and Hilda both described severe cases:

VIRGINIA: I saw people with diabetes going into eye clinic who had cataracts, who had glaucoma, and I would see the patches on their eyes, I would see them with canes, I just never thought these were other people that I saw, it wasn't until it got to my dad and my grandparents and, that I realized how bad it can become. I had a grandfather on my mother's side and he, I know he had missing fingers he had I think it was his whole right, his left hand where all of his fingers were gone. I just knew that as a kid growing up, I didn't know why. I thought maybe just he had an accident. He had diabetes and he had his fingers amputated because of diabetes. And you know just when I realized it was because of diabetes it started to scare me and so knowing that I'm already heavyset. [thirty-one-year-old Navajo woman with diabetic family members]

HILDA: He ended up in the hospital where we almost lost him, that's severe, yeah, that's what I call severe, I mean, you know for him to fall over at work and they say he was in a coma for a little while there because he was so bad off and he didn't know what was going on, he was in and out and stuff, so that's a severe one. [fifty-three-year-old Meskwaki woman with diabetic family members]

As described earlier, there is a moralizing discourse about diabetes care in the community. In cases of severe diabetes, moralizing discussions of patient care are more pointed. Community members expect that those who have suffered complications of diabetes will care for the disease more closely to avoid further complications—and these care expectations most often focus on consumption. One day while in the center kitchen preparing for senior lunch, a center staff member told me of an elder community member who was admitted to the hospital for her diabetes. This elder had already suffered diabetes complications, and the staff member informed me that her daughter had found some empty cans of regular soda and candy wrappers in the trash. The staff member described this elder's consumption as reckless, and particularly so because she had already lost several toes.

Diabetes in Native Chicago is understood and organized by a local system of classification that has been shaped by what community members observe in cases of the disease among family and friends. These classifications shape behavior and discourses, not only of the individual living with diabetes but of others in the community who interact with diabetics. This emic model differs from the etic model found in biomedical literature in significant ways. First, it is primarily focused on type 2 and borderline cases of diabetes. Second, it is organized around the types of care intervention used to treat the condition. Individual experiences with treating the condition are shared in informal conversations; the emic classification system is both developed and upheld through these discussions, of which the kitchen conversation about the community elder who was admitted to the hospital is a poignant example.

In this chapter I have shown that diabetes is prevalent in Native Chicago, a prevalence that shapes local understandings and conceptions of the disease. Children are aware of its existence and sometimes of the related care needs at a young age. Due to the already high rate of diabetes in the community and the public health sector's labeling of Indigenous Americans as at risk for developing the condition, fatalistic views about diabetes development abound. While there is little stigma surrounding the development of diabetes, there is moralizing discussion of the care acts of others. Furthermore, the community describes diabetes along a spectrum, defining the disease from mild to severe cases based upon the treatment needs and the effect the condition has on individual lives. In the next chapter I take a step back and look more closely at definitions of diabetes itself and local explanations for why there are high rates of this disease in Native communities, both in cities and on reservations.

5

Local Understandings and Explanations of Diabetes

With a digital voice recorder lying between us in my black Honda Civic, we exited Lake Shore Drive onto Wilson Avenue, making our way to the American Indian Center. Rebecca kept an eye out for community members she knows as we drove down the street through heavy pedestrian traffic. We were nearing the end of our shared commute that warm June morning, and I had one more question for Rebecca before we arrived at our destination—why do people develop diabetes?

> REBECA: My reasoning, and I mean my mom thought the same thing, 'cause . . . well, her family, my mom's family, they don't have diabetes. But they lived on the farm, they had their horses, their cattle, everything that they grew or farmed their own. But the ones that lived in Macy [Nebraska] relied on the commodities, the food that the government handed out . . . I don't think Native people, their bodies, it was just introduced a few generations ago, all the sugars and everything else . . . Native bodies just can't adapt to it. [fifty-three-year-old Odawa/Omaha woman]

Her response mirrors the explanations given by other interviewees; Native people and Native bodies are not accustomed to eating the diet brought by setters into the Americas, and this has led to a susceptibility to developing diabetes.

In this chapter I explore how conceptions of diabetes are situated within the experience and care for diabetes in Native Chicago and how these discourses offer a look into local world views on evolution, colonial history, and Native identity. In the first section, I show that local diabetes definitions are varied and situated within personal experiences with the disease. In the second, I document local explanations for diabetes with a focus on explanations for high rates of diabetes in Indigenous American populations. Local explanations, I demonstrate, not only offer local understandings of diabetes etiology but also strengthen notions of a shared Native identity in this urban space through discussions of shared history and shared bodies. The separation of diabetes definitions from explanations is an arbitrary one I employ to organize this chapter, and, as will become apparent, there is great overlap in explanations and definitions for diabetes in local discourse.

Defining Diabetes in Native Chicago

In chapter 3 I described how the current biomedical model defines diabetes as being characterized by hyperglycemia due to insulin resistance or deficiency. Though there is not a clear understanding as to why people develop the disease, genes and environment are described in this model as two of the most influential factors in diabetes etiology. The biomedical model focuses on the disease on some of the smaller levels within the human body. While influenced by this paradigm, local definitions of diabetes in Native Chicago focus on the experience of the condition in individual and social life. Local definitions vary, corresponding with different life experiences.

Individual experiences with the biomedical model of diabetes encountered in clinical appointments, in informational print materials like pamphlets, and in group education settings like the American Indian Health Service of Chicago's Diabetes Talking Circle series influence local definitions of the disease. This influence is seen in frequently encountered discussions of blood sugar, pancreas, and insulin:

LESTER: You know diabetes is just that your body's not producing enough insulin. [fifty-eight-year-old Sioux/white man living with diabetes]

CHRISTY: Your body doesn't produce enough insulin, so basically that causes your blood sugar to be very high because your body doesn't produce enough insulin so you develop diabetes. [thirty-three-year-old Ojibwe woman with diabetic family members]

LOIS: Diabetes is a, I think it's where your pancreas doesn't make no insulin or we take in sugar and we can't, it can't dissolve it or it can't get it out of your body, so we do it by going to the bathroom a lot too. It's, that's one other thing, we pee a lot, you know trying to get the sugar flow. We got to drink a lot of water to get it flushed out of our system. So it's, it's, it creates problems if we don't get the insulin to you. [fifty-eight-year-old Ojibwe woman living with diabetes]

TIFFANY: Like if my daughter was to ask me, I would tell her that it's the sugars that are in your body they can't be broken down, they get too high and everything has to be even in your body in order for it to you know give you off the energy and stuff like that and I'd let her know it's just from eating too much sweet stuff and you know. [thirty-nine-year-old Seneca woman with diabetic family members]

These local definitions share attributes with the biomedical model. Diabetes is described here as a problem within the body. Tiffany refers to the latter being unable to break down food—here offering a response to her eleven-year-old daughter's hypothetical question about what diabetes is. While Lois locates the failure in the pancreas, she joins Lester and Christy in referring to it as a lack of insulin.

The incorporation of institutionalized medical understandings of health and disease into lay models of disease is common in populations worldwide. Linda Hunt's work on cancer in southern Mexico demonstrates that understandings of cancer in this setting are influenced both by local experiences and expectations and by bio-medical models.[1] As mentioned previously, Puneet Chawla Sahota's work in a southwestern Indigenous American reservation commu-nity describes the continuing influence the thrifty genotype hypoth-esis has on contemporary understandings of diabetes.[2] At the same time, while institutionalized medical models influence understand-ings of human health and disease, the definition of disease in local communities is also greatly influenced by personal experience.[3] In her work with a Canadian Ojibwe community, Linda Garro demon-strates that diabetes is understood through personal experience and encounters with the condition.[4] Through personal and social encounters with disease and disease care, local models of disease diverge from institutionalized models, in some cases significantly. For instance, Susan McCombie shows that common illnesses like "the flu" can be understood differently by biomedically trained epi-demiologists and the lay public: namely, the lay public more com-monly understands "the flu" to refer to a gastrointestinal condition, whereas epidemiologists see "the flu" as referring to a respiratory illness.[5] Local diabetes definitions in Native Chicago mirror some aspects of the biomedical definition of the disease but are also being shaped by personal experiences with the disease and its care.

People experience diabetes in different ways. According to partic-ipants living with the disease in this study, some feel no symptoms when their blood glucose level is elevated, while others describe cases of polydipsia, polyuria, having wounds that will not heal, blurred vision, and feeling dizzy, fatigued, hyper, and/or weak. Lois's definition of diabetes quoted above refers to the experi-ences of polyuria and polydipsia. Sylvia, who has been living with diabetes for six years, defined the disease only by its symptoms:

SYLVIA: I'd say you have to use the bathroom all the time, you're thirsty and losing weight. [sixty-nine-year-old Chippewa woman]

The symptoms of diabetes experienced in the day-to-day life of people living with it and caring for it factor prominently into their definitions of the condition.

In addition to symptoms of hyperglycemia, people define diabetes with reference to the work that is required for its care. Physicians recommend diabetics manage the disease by testing blood glucose levels, following a diet plan that typically limits the amount of carbohydrates consumed at dedicated mealtimes, increasing daily physical activity, and/or taking oral medications or injections of insulin. Colin, a nineteen-year-old Cherokee man, described that developing diabetes in early adulthood has been particularly difficult because of the restrictions the disease has placed on his life:

COLIN: My explanation to that would be a very very bad disease to have. It don't allow you to eat the things you want to. You got to constantly check your blood sugar. Just really nonsense, especially if you're a kid. It's worse with sisters and stuff. It's not something that you would like to have at a young age.

Having diabetes in youth and early adulthood is difficult because the disease separates Colin from his age mates—he has to manage his blood glucose and be cautious of his food intake while out with friends who do not share these restrictions. Further, it is hard for him while still living at home with younger sisters, whom he describes as taunting him by "rubbing their candy in [his] face." These markers of disease separate young diabetics in the community from nondiabetic family and friends and can thwart care efforts—a topic I discuss in more detail in the following chapter.

Care requirements factor into definitions of diabetes for patients and caregivers of all ages:

ARIA: It's having to do something you don't want to do. Having it, I guess, it's having something that can control the rest of your life if you can't control it. You don't want something that controls you. And that's just pretty much what it does if you don't get the strength to do what you're supposed to, which I'm finding out. [thirty-four-year-old Assiniboine woman living with diabetes]

PHILLIP: A crippling disease you know that you could avoid by watching diet and exercising, you know and checking in with your doctor you know. And watching your diet and keeping up on it, you know, monitoring. [fifty-two-year-old Micmac man living with diabetes]

LYLE: Oh, diabetes is an invasion. I mean it's just an invasion on your life. I mean a life that you, it's just an invasion on your life and an impact, the impact from that is, it's crazy. It's really crazy. For me it is anyways, because to me diabetes is just, it's an invasion on your whole life, it's just that's the way it is. [forty-seven-year-old Menominee/Ho-Chunk man with diabetic family members]

Diabetes is referred to by those living with and helping care for the condition as "very very bad," "an invasion," "crippling," "crazy," "nonsense," and "something that can control the rest of your life if you can't control it." The experience of caring for and living with diabetes in daily life is central to defining the disease. The entire life of the person and their family and friends is altered by the requirements of diabetes management.

As discussed in the last chapter, people learn and know through engagement in the world, and this is the case with medical knowledge. For example, ethnographer Annemarie Mol describes how physicians, lab technicians, and other health-care workers within one Dutch hospital hold widely different understandings of atherosclerosis. Mol shows that there are multiple ontologies of atherosclerosis based upon the perspective of actors in different departments in this hospital. The understanding each actor has of the condition is dependent upon the type of engagement they have with it. In the clinic, atherosclerosis is a disease that causes pain while walking, in the hematologist's laboratory it is a blood disease, and in the pathology laboratory it is the thickening of the vein walls.[6] Similarly, definitions of diabetes in Native Chicago are situated within individual, social, and dialogical experiences with the disease—from those first observations made in childhood to the experiences later in life of developing and/or caring for the daily management of the condition. In Native Chicago, local community members not only witness diabetes care routines from a young age but also become familiar with serious health complications associated with "severe" cases. Native Chicagoans incorporate these diabetes complications and the effect they have on individuals and on the community into their definitions:

NATALIE: Diabetes is a killer that's all I can say . . . just from my own experiences growing up, and I saw that all my life. I saw some horrific things and it scared me. [sixty-eight-year-old Ottawa woman with diabetic family members]

BOBBIE: It's your sugar levels and how you eat, if you don't eat right, then your sugar levels are going to go sky high and you could be blind, which my girlfriend . . . she went blind for two weeks and she did not know she was a diabetic, even though it runs in the family. She went to the hospital, she goes, well I can't see. And they took her to the hospital, she got it down to where it should but she never knew she was diabetic. And one of my boyfriends I used to date, he now lives on the reservation in Wisconsin. He lost his, he's losing his eyesight, his legs are giving out from being a diabetic and his sister too. She lives here and she's a diabetic. She got one of her toes cut off, so as soon as I found out that, I thought well I'm taking my pills, I'm not going to be. You never know, your kidneys, one of the girls, my girlfriend's friend used to live next door, her neighbor, her kidneys failed because she was a diabetic, so anything can happen. [fifty-two-year-old Chippewa woman living with diabetes]

Local definitions of diabetes are, as Natalie described, built upon what people have seen and experienced as part of their individual lifeworld. These experiences shape understandings of the disease, and as Bobbie described, influence personal care practices.

In chapter 4 I described how fatalistic views of diabetes are widespread in Chicago's Native community. Some community members incorporate this fatalism into their definitions of diabetes, referring to diabetes as a socially accepted disease. Virginia explains:

VIRGINIA: I would say diabetes is a lifelong condition that you really want to keep away from being diagnosed for yourself or a family member or even a friend, because diabetes affects your life in a drastic, drastic way that people are not aware of. They are not aware of the ramifications of the individual and the person that are nearby the close, the loved ones, how it affects them physically, emotionally, you know, just in all aspects. It's, it seems, and it seems like diabetes, it seems to be in everyday thing, but it's just become so so common that people have just forgotten about it. And I think everyone needs to [be] reeducated on the severity of the causes of diabetes and what diabetes can do to a person. [thirty-one-year-old Navajo woman with diabetic family members]

Here, the ubiquity of the disease creates a sense of normalcy about diabetes in the community. This "normality," both she and another interviewee named Barry contend, endangers Chicago's Native community and its future health and well-being. In an unrecorded interview, Barry explained that "diabetes is not a hereditary thing, but a socially accepted thing that makes you sick." Barry went on to explain that people are eating the wrong types of food and in great quantity. While Virginia and Barry describe diabetes as socially accepted, they promote increased education and prevention of the disease, particularly for younger generations.

Diabetes is defined in Chicago's Native community in several ways. These definitions are formed through life experiences—including attending biomedical appointments, reading print and electronic sources on diabetes, experiencing diabetes symptoms, caring for the disease, and witnessing family and community experiences with diabetes care and complications.

Local Explanations for Diabetes Development

In Holly's explanation for why Native populations have high rates of diabetes (in the introduction to this book) and in Tiffany's definition of diabetes as the body's inability to break down food, the body's ability to metabolize food is central to diabetes definitions. In his definition of diabetes, Charles, the Sioux man described in chapter 4 as supporting eating the diet of one's ancestors, offered a definition of diabetes from a slightly different vantage point, describing diabetes as a problem with specific types of food rather than with Native bodies:

> CHARLES: I define diabetes to be an allergic reaction to sugar, sugary foods, like starchy foods, high starchy foods. I don't believe that everyone should be consuming complex carbohydrates and a lot of sugar. It should be minimal. It should be a minimal part of Native Americans' diets as we live. We have a sensitivity to a lot of different foods and you know sugar being one. That's why I would, that's why I would guess that, that we're just not, I guess you could say programmed to eat that kind of a diet. [thirty-one-year-old Sioux man with diabetic family members]

Rather than focusing on the individual body as the site of disease, Charles's definition focused on the contemporary American diet—a diet he describes as high in starch and sugar. As noted earlier, Charles saw diabetes as a set of diseases falling along a spectrum of sensitivity to this new diet. Over the millennia before settler arrival, the Indigenous peoples of the Americas evolved to eat a certain type of diet that was severely restricted or taken away through colonialism. Native bodies are not accustomed to eating this new diet, which, for Charles, explains why Native populations have begun to develop diabetes in recent decades.

Biomedical researchers are still seeking for an explanation as to why people first develop diabetes. Contemporary mainstream biomedical models focus on genetics and environmental factors. In this section I look at the discourses on diabetes causation in Native Chicago. I show that while these explanations offer reasoning for why people develop diabetes, they further highlight and support notions of shared Native history and physiology that contribute to conceptions of Native identity and community in this city space. Two less commonly cited biomedical explanations for diabetes development are discussed here—stress and transgenerational epigenetics—where they correspond with local models for diabetes development.

Inheritance

In Bobbie's discussion of diabetes complications quoted above, she described a girlfriend of hers who lost her vision for a period due to diabetes she did not even know she had. Bobbie implied that the friend ought to have known earlier, noting that the disease "runs in her family." In other words, diabetes is considered an inherited disease in Native Chicago. Inheritance in this context is a complicated subject, as has been found in other locales. Inheritance can refer to genetic inheritance, family inheritance, blood inheritance, and inheritance of social behaviors and customs. In her research with Native communities in Arizona and southern California, Diane Weiner found that the description of diabetes as an inherited disease can be confounded in local interpretations. In this setting she found that doctors refer to diabetes as an inherited trait when speaking with patients. Weiner explains that the physicians in this case are referring to genetic inheritance, but their patients most often understand inheritance to be a social legacy of lifestyle—such as the diet they eat.[7] As explained in chapter 3, local biomedical providers interviewed for the present study describe diabetes as both a genetically and socially inherited condition—referring particularly to an inheritance of eating customs and socioeconomic situations that shape and limit lifestyle options.

The diabetes epidemic among America's Indigenous populations has been linked to a hypothetical thrifty genotype, and while biomedical researchers have argued against this explanation for diabetes development, the idea of the thrifty genotype has lasting power in conversations about the disease in reservation spaces. Sahota finds that community members on a southwestern reservation incorporate local understandings of the thrifty genotype hypothesis into their accounts of diabetes.[8] The genotype in this context is understood as a type of survival gene that was once beneficial, but which in contemporary times interferes with the body's ability to process modern diets. The thrifty genotype hypothesis was not referenced by interviewees in Native Chicago. However, the idea of a specifically Native American body that evolved to live and prosper in the environment of North America is widely shared and present in local discussions of diabetes.

The idea of diabetes as genetically inherited or passed down in the physical makeup from one generation to the next was a common feature in diabetes explanations I encountered. I noted that Chris described the likelihood of all his siblings developing diabetes in the section on fatalistic views of diabetes in the previous chapter. This view was based upon Chris's conception of diabetes as a genetically transmitted trait:

> CHRIS: My younger sister doesn't have it yet. She's lucky. I don't know why, maybe she diets too much or something. But we, I never, you know I never ate a lot of sweets either. I don't, so I don't know why I got diabetes. They said it's like from eating sugar. But I don't eat sugar a lot. I think it's in, with me, it's my genes. [forty-five-year-old Potawatomi/Puerto Rican man living with diabetes]

Chris recognized that many other people attribute diabetes to diet and exercise, but he found this explanation inadequate for his case, seeing it as a condition passed down the family line through genes.

Inheritance can refer to many things. In Native Chicago, diabetes was described to me as inherited genetically, through blood lines, through family lines, and through social means. Idella, quoted in the introduction to chapter 4, questioned whether diabetes was in Native blood. This link between blood inheritance and diabetes was commonly cited by community members, as was the idea that diabetes "runs in families":

> ESTHER: My mom always told me that I have to watch out for that because it runs in both sides of my family. [nineteen-year-old Ojibwe woman with diabetic family members]

> TAMMY: It ran in our families. [sixty-eight-year-old Oneida woman living with diabetes]

Native Chicagoans link diabetes to both physical and social forms of inheritance. While the biomedical providers described in chapter 3 consider social inheritance of dietary habits as a primary factor in the increased diabetes rates for this population, community members more often refer to colonial history when discussing the role of diet in diabetes development.

Colonialism, Diet, and Poverty

Life conditions are an important factor in understandings of diabetes causation in Native Chicago. Roy explained that while there are a lot of pieces that factor into why people develop diabetes, food is the primary cause:

ROY: Diabetes comes from many different things. I mean the majority of it is from the food that we consume. [thirty-five-year-old Oglala Sioux/Navajo man with diabetic family members]

In chapter 3 I discussed the work of Lorelei de Cora, Yvonne Jackson, Betty Geishirt Cantrell, and James Justice, which posits that the contemporary diabetes epidemic in Native populations can be attributed to the recent diet changes brought on by colonialism. Indeed, many members of Chicago's Native community see colonialism as continuing to exist in the present, as their homeland is inhabited by settlers. In a collaborative work on diabetes in Ojibwe and Dakota communities, Linda Garro and Gretchen Chesley Lang describe that some individuals relate the disease to diet, specifically to the consumption of too much sugar, while others see a strong association between diabetes and the movement away from traditional Ojibwe and Dakota practices.[9] In a similar vein, Devon Abbott Mihesuah's book *Recovering Our Ancestors' Gardens* advocates returning to ancestral lifeways, as a means both of achieving food sovereignty and improving well-being.[10]

In Native Chicago, colonial history factors significantly into discussions of why people began to develop diabetes. Steven, quoted in chapter 3 as explaining that Natives did not encounter diseases like diabetes prior to contact with settler communities, continued his historical account of Indigenous American diabetes development:

STEVEN: These people came and they cleared the land and killed everything that was on the land. Okay, now the Indians don't have anything to eat. Here's all these white people settlers' colonies coming in. Okay, now what are they going to do? These Indians are starving, did they go and live off the colonists and they start eating all this stuff that they eat? And that's the start right there, that's, that's my philosophy, but that's, that's what I think is because that they. You know back in their day, they were the healthiest people, you know what I mean, it's like in, and now, and like I said, I've read in some books where they, even the elders tell them, you know the reason things are so bad is because you, you've gone away from your cultures and your original way your people were, the way you did things, the way you farmed, the way you prepared your foods, you're, it's all, the white man's come with metal pots, you used to use all these old wooden bowls and stuff where you never, you never used the white man's things, now you got all these white man's comforts and all this stuff, you know. [sixty-one-year-old Seneca man living with diabetes]

As argued earlier, diabetes must be understood in the social and historical context; colonialism forced diet and other life condition changes that resulted in the Indigenous American diabetes epidemic. Today, societal structures of poverty, racism, and social marginalization play a role in the continuation of this situation, thwarting prevention measures and inhibiting capabilities for improved care and management. As Steven described, even though historically Indigenous Americans "were the healthiest people," changes to diet and life conditions have resulted in increased cases of diabetes (along with cancer, depression, and obesity), such that over these few centuries, Natives shifted from one of the "healthiest" populations to a population that suffers some of the worst health outcomes in a nation characterized by serious health disparities.[11]

Local explanations for diabetes include not only these diet changes but also the poverty of life conditions. Tammy lived on the Oneida reservation until her early twenties and attributed her development of diabetes at the age of twenty-nine to her diet in that context:

> TAMMY: When I was growing up on the reservation, we ate whatever we could, whatever there was for us to eat. I mean 'cause we were very poor, so. You know nowadays, you know naturally quite a lot of people work so their food and diets are a little bit better. But at that time we, like I said, we ate what we, what was put on the table in front of us. [sixty-eight-year-old Oneida woman living with diabetes]

Poverty and the political economy of food—the political and economic components organizing the distribution and accessibility of food—continue to factor into diabetes explanations in urban spaces.[12]

Debbie, a forty-seven-year-old Ho-Chunk woman with diabetic family members explained that diabetes affects socioeconomic classes differently in the city:

> DEBBIE: I think poverty plays a big role in it too, because not everybody has the right foods to eat, so poverty plays a big role in a lot of things. You know I know a lot of people who eat organic, now I can't friggin' afford organic, no I can't afford no friggin' organic. You wonder why all these movie stars and everybody's so healthy and all this other stuff is because they had the means and the ways to hire this you know whatever the hell to get in shape and dietician and yeah. You have to have the means and the ways to you know, to eat right.

In Native Chicago, social and economic status is considered a factor for diabetes development, one that works its way particularly into discussions of diet and exercise. Specifically, the diabetes epidemic has been related to the change in diet from precolonial diets to diets high in fat and simple carbohydrates like sugar and white flour.[13] In the city the dietary explanation takes on a particular color due to the urban context. The political economy of food is considered by community members as a contributing factor to poor health. People describe the need for meals that are quick to make, relatively inexpensive, and filling enough to keep them going through their workday, commute, school, and taking care of children. In Native Chicago, the cost of food is the primary concern, and not only cost in terms of financial cost: the cost of time is also an important consideration. Foods that are convenient and require little preparation are common. People frequently turn to fast food restaurants that are easily accessible in the city, or to premade or easy to make meals found in grocery stores; these are inexpensive and have high carbohydrate, fat, sugar, and sodium content. Based on responses to the surveys collected in 2015 for this study, 20.4 percent of this population reports an income that is considered below the 2015 national poverty line based on household size. Another 38.8 percent are living on the border of the poverty line, with incomes just one to five thousand dollars above the poverty threshold for their household size.

Complicating matters, some community health-care workers associate diabetes in this community with the social inheritance of eating habits. Though the staff at the American Indian Center strives to serve foods that are considered healthier, the health-care workers describe food at center events as concerning. While the American Indian Center had a dietician on staff, sodium, carbohydrates, and portion sizes were closely monitored for elder lunches. In more recent years, staff continue to consider these factors but will often provide second portions of food to those who ask for more, effectively doubling the intake for one meal. Staff members explain that they are concerned with when and where some community members will get their next meal. In the 2015 surveys, nearly 42 percent of respondents reported that they had experienced food insecurity in their lifetime, not knowing when or where they would get their next meal. The experience of food insecurity shapes the cooking, serving, and eating habits at community events. It is this response to these concerns that worries health-care workers who did not grow up in the community. As non-Native community health-care provider Cheryl describes:

CHERYL: They're great cooks, you know, and the food's good, and they just like, they pile it on. And that was one of my big discoveries. I mean to me it was a big discovery, was that really the feast or famine thing is still there. You know it's like eat all you can 'cause who knows where the next meal is going to be from, you know, and you would hear that at different gatherings. [sixty-three-year-old non-Native nurse]

The uncertainty of food supply in the not-so-distant past for many and in the present for some shapes contemporary eating habits.

Stress

Stress is described as another factor influencing both diabetes development and care in Native Chicago. Pauline explains that the stress of trying to "make ends meet" living in Chicago played a role in her diabetes. Pauline raised her own two children and six foster children while working in the city. When she was laid off two years before our interview, she lost not only her income but her home. Stress caused by financial burdens and work life were cited as factors in the development of diabetes in Native Chicago by several interviewees, and these external pressures also played a role in shaping diabetes management.

Psychological stress is described as a factor in diabetes causation in communities worldwide. In Gretchen Chesley Lang's work on Dakota understandings of diabetes' causes, she finds that here diabetes is related to diet, to loss of tradition, and to increased levels of psychological stress.[14] Melanie Rock also finds that Cree individuals describe a strong association of diabetes with both distress and duress.[15] This focus on the relationship of diabetes, emotions, and stress in patient perspectives is seen in other cultural contexts outside of Indigenous American populations. In a 1988 study medical anthropologist Jo Scheder argues that growing cases of diabetes among migrant workers appear to be closely associated with high levels of stress.[16] Jane Poss and Mary Jezewski describe how Mexican patients they interviewed considered *susto* (fear) to be a causal factor, along with diet and obesity.[17] Samantha Thompson and Sandra Gifford describe that members of the Aboriginal community they work with attribute diabetes to "being out of balance."[18] Steve Ferzacca's study of health and healing in modern Java describes how community members associate modern ailments like diabetes with the newly developed urban condition of *stres* (stress).[19] In their study of Mexican American patients living in Chicago, Emily Mendenhall and colleagues find that their respondents often saw stress as a significant factor in their diabetes development; indeed, for some, diabetes was considered the embodiment of stress.[20] Similarly, Nancy Schoenberg and colleagues find that diabetes patients from African American, Indigenous American, Mexican American, and rural white American communities in the United States believe that stress not only contributes to the development of diabetes but can also exacerbate the condition and hinder one's ability to manage the disease.[21] So strong does the correlation between stress and diabetes appear to be that it has been included in the biomedical model of the disease.

The inclusion of stress as a possible causal factor for diabetes in medical models began in the seventeenth century. Thomas Willis, who contributed to the disease's classification by adding mellitus to the nomenclature *diabetes mellitus* in recognition of the sweetness of a diabetic patient's urine, included in his description of the disease the hypothesis that an overconsumption of ale as well as extended periods of sorrow contribute to its development.[22] Willis's inclusion of psychological distress has gained further support in the past few decades of biomedical research on the factors contributing to diabetes etiology. For example, Per Björntorp argues that perceived stress results in an activation of the hypothalamic-pituitary-adrenal axis, increased levels of cortisol production, and reduced amounts of sex hormones; these reactions, Björntorp explains, contribute to the buildup of visceral fat, which along with increased levels of cortisol is associated with insulin resistance, thus creating a link between stress and diabetes.[23] Pickup and Crook postulate a role for the innate immune system in diabetes development. In their hypothesis, stress-induced sustained activity of the immune system results in an increased secretion of cytokines, cell-signaling protein molecules. These increased cytokines are then linked to the release of proteins and hormones from the liver, the adipose tissue, and the brain. Pickup and Crook explain that these released hormones and proteins are associated with insulin resistance; in their model, if a person is already predisposed to developing diabetes through family history or environmental factors, the innate immune system may play a role in the development of diabetes through reactions to stress.[24]

Local and biomedical views of stress and how it might factor into diabetes differ in terms of perspective. In local explanations, people define stress both in emotional and psychological terms. In recent studies of the role of stress in diabetes development, biomedical models focus on the physiological effects both emotional and psychosocial stress have on bodies, looking at hormone production as a factor in creating insulin resistant cells. While these perspectives differ in the particulars, both local and biomedical researchers consider life stress a possible factor contributing to diabetes development.

Intergenerational Trauma

Intergenerational trauma is increasingly gaining attention in Native American health research. Community health worker Dacia offered a definition of the concept from her own experience growing up in Native Chicago and now working in the health-care field:

> DACIA: Our families are hurting. Our families, like whole entire units of families are in pain. And we don't really fully understand always what that pain is about. We just know that we're hurting. And, but it's not depression. Well, I should say community isn't exactly viewed as depression, because I'm not feeling like I want to kill myself. So they're not being able to recognize this form of

depression and so I'm living my life and I have my family and we're moving day to day and we're getting it done. We're getting it done on a bare minimum kind of scale. It's not a full functioning, it's not fully functional and operational, because we're just, we're running on zero constantly and you recharge only enough to make it through the next day . . .

And a lot of it our families aren't talking about it. So we have families that have been hurt for whatever reason from, you know, two generations ago, they never talked about it. We know whatever secrets lie in, in grandma's closet, but we don't talk about it. Those are secrets that continue to remain secrets and you know about it, but we're not going to go there. And then now those same things are being, are occurring to us in some, maybe it's the same manner or similar manner or you know whatever. It's just a different scenery, different people involved, but there's the same things that are happening because nobody is teaching us how to talk it out. Instead it's like you have to bury it deep down inside ourselves and pretend that I'm good, I'm fine . . .

We learn to put on a smiling face, and we learn to bury those things deep down, and we don't know how to, you know, so we learn to do those kinds of things and we can present as, no, I'm normal, and then it's like, okay we're waiting, we're waiting, she's going to look away, whew. [forty-one-year-old Oneida community health worker]

Intergenerational trauma is trauma that is passed from one generation to the next. As Dacia described, this trauma is not just felt by community members in Native Chicago, it is performed—in this case by having to wear a smile to mask the hurt. Many events and policies in colonial history factor into local discussions of intergenerational trauma, including the boarding school system, forced removal to reservations, and individual events like the massacres at Wounded Knee and Sand Creek.

The concept of intergenerational trauma as a factor influencing Native health is moving from the biomedical community to local communities. In Native Chicago, depression and intergenerational trauma are widely believed to be closely related. In the fields of psychology and social medicine, intergenerational trauma is referred to as historical trauma. This concept was developed in the 1990s as a way of looking at the intersection of historical oppression and psychological trauma, with the important recognition that historical events impact contemporary wellness, even spanning multiple generations.[25]

Dacia does not link the development of diabetes to intergenerational trauma, though some of her colleagues in the Native health-care community do believe there is a link, an understanding shared by some within the community itself. For example, Charles described:

> CHARLES: Well I would say that it's a combination of things. It's not, it's such a problem where you can't just point to one, one thing and then say that's the problem. I think that there are several things . . . I also feel that there's a cultural, it's a matter of historical trauma. People have, people who have gone through, just about every one of us has family members and grandparents who have gone through the boarding school system and I believe just like with alcohol, there's a lot of depression that people had experienced as we've had our whole, our whole two or three generations of parents and grandparents have been you know pretty much wiped out and in a sense brainwashed so there was like not a lot of, so the parenting you know, they didn't understand how to be parents because they were taught that what they were was what was wrong with the world, you know, they taught them worse things, they taught them to hate themselves and in turn they hated who they were and then their kids grew up hating themselves and just be a cycle, a whole cycle of, of very unstable households because you know it's this different understanding, they lost a lot of their teachings, so I believe that that's definitely a factor as well. [thirty-one-year-old Sioux man with diabetic family members]

Charles was the only community member who described intergenerational trauma as a factor in the development of diabetes. Others spoke of the relationship between intergenerational trauma and depression and alcoholism in the community, a topic I return to in the next chapter in discussing diabetes management practices.

While community members did not often speak of diabetes as being caused by intergenerational trauma, nurses who have worked in the community for long periods of time, including the former wellness director of the American Indian Center Laura, describe it as a contributing factor to diabetes etiology in this community. Carla, a twenty-four-year-old Native/white nurse, explained:

> CARLA: I think it had a lot, it has a lot to do with, it's kind of a multitude of factors in terms of poverty, historically just coming from being, I think it has to do with historical trauma, poverty and kind of how we treat food now versus the way we used to . . . People should definitely, people are kind of starting to talk about it more in terms of relation to health care and it should be, definitely. Because you know it's, it could be just poverty as well, I mean if you look at other poverty, regions with extreme poverty they have obesity, diabetes, things like that as well. But that, then also, then their poverty they have historical trauma too. It's a lot to do with a lot of Native family, families have [a] multitude of social issues, I feel like carry on, you know there's abuse, there's stress, there's broken homes, different things like that. You can't really raise healthy children if you don't live in a healthy mental environment and that cycle just kind of continues you know broken home leads to maybe that person having a broken home in the future with their family, so I feel like we definitely have a lot to do with it.

The role of transgenerational epigenetics is an area of interest that has grown in biomedical sciences in recent decades and corresponds to these local discussions of intergenerational trauma. The field studies the passage of cell information between generations that is not encoded in DNA. Michael Skinner and colleagues posit that environmentally induced changes to epigenetic elements—

including DNA methylation, histone modifications, chromatin structure, and hydroxymethylcytosine residues in the brain—can persist and be inherited by the next generation.[26] Though human studies are limited (in contrast to animal studies), researchers find that one generation's experience of stress leading to neuroendocrine responses affect not only that generation but subsequent generations. Stephen Matthews and David Phillips describe that this passage has an effect on the hypothalamic-pituitary-adrenal axis, causing hypercortisolemia, which, as described above, can lead to insulin resistance, as well as depression and hypertension.[27] Transgenerational epigenetics is a burgeoning area of research that offers support to the argument that intergenerational trauma may play a role in diabetes development.

Local explanations for why people develop diabetes concern a wide range of factors that include family inheritance, diet, colonial history, stress, and intergenerational trauma. Local understandings of diabetes etiology, like biomedical explanations, describe diabetes development as complex and multifaceted. Diabetes is typically described as being caused by several of these factors together. As described in chapter 3, the mainstream biomedical model for diabetes focuses on locating the cause for disease within the internal structures of individual bodies. The role that sociopolitical histories play in the development of conditions like diabetes should be earnestly considered in discussions of disease etiology. For America's Indigenous population, the current diabetes epidemic is the embodiment of colonial and structural violence.

Native Identity and Community in Discourses of Diabetes

These local discourses not only offer explanations for why people develop diabetes—they further provide a window into local worldviews about Native identity, group membership, and colonial history. In local explanations and definitions of diabetes, there is an underlying discourse that speaks to local conceptions of Native identity, community, history, evolution, and race. Natives of all Indigenous nations in these discussions are described as sharing a similar body, developed over millennia. In this discourse Native and former Native diets are described as "good," "natural," and "pure" and contrasted with the diets of modern America, which are seen as a significant factor in the diabetes epidemic among Native populations today.

Several interlocutors shared these ideas in interviews, highlighting their articulation within local understandings of diabetes development. Below, I cite a few of these conversations, including the statement from Holly that opened this book:

HOLLY: One of the things that I think of in our diets that our bodies aren't used to as Native people is that the settlers brought, the government brought, gave us white products—the salt, the sugar, the flour, dairy, all those things were things our bodies weren't used to, and they each took a toll and, you know some of those things together or separate, however you want to say it, came in the form of bringing diabetes . . . I think the bodies aren't able to process it. I think that Native people are used to very natural diets where they ate off the land, they ate grains, they drank teas from the earth. Everything was very simple and very pure. [forty-four-year-old Apache/Sioux woman with diabetic family members]

ROSANNA: I think of it like historically, like our food systems were ripped from our people, so federally mandated that, kill all of the bison. And they were almost completely decimated. I think there's plant colonization, so people brought their different plants from whatever countries they were coming from and that either you know adversely affected plant life that was here or whatever it may be, introduction of, like, pig and cow and chicken. Those are not our natural foods. Frybread as traditional as it may seem today, that was really just Native people being adaptive at a time when they were, you know, kept on reservations taken away from their foods systems and then only given federally mandated flour and oil and the government was feeding us foods that were not ours and our systems were kind of in a shock. Our systems are still in a shock reaction from that. [twenty-eight-year-old Oneida woman with diabetic family members]

LOIS: We had a pure system. We weren't, we weren't, we were not accustomed to these, to all this sugar and all these products that were, that everyone else was. Natives had a system where they only had natural, so all this other stuff that was, that we had is unnatural to us, and so our bodies are not adjusted to it ... Maybe down the line, maybe our systems will adjust to it, but right now we're still in the pure. We're still in the pure system. [fifty-eight-year-old Ojibwe woman living with diabetes]

MONICA: You know, I mean I get down to like the basic, like back in the day when the government put the Natives on the reservation and gave them these certain foods to eat and we had to figure out how to use these things to feed our families, which those weren't a part of our life. It was all, you know the wild rices, the good beef, you know, the buffalo, and the deer, and the rabbits, you know, the good things, and the roots and everything that really was with our tradition and our culture for centuries before. So I think that played a lot to do with it. [forty-four-year-old Sioux/Ponca woman living with diabetes]

Chicago's intertribal community is strengthened through these discourses of not only a shared social and political history of displacement and oppression but also a shared evolutionary history that is embodied today through the experiences of diabetes in Native communities. In chapter 2 I described how a shared history of colonial oppression is referenced in local discussions of Native identity in the city. In these diabetes discourses, Native identity is defined in terms of a history predating colonialism—a shared evolutionary history that produced bodies that hunger for pure and natural foods and are susceptible to diabetes today.

In these discussions, the health of the social and the individual body correspond with group membership. In Native Chicago, a vulnerability to diabetes is a widely recognized characteristic of Indigenous populations of North America. To be an Indigenous American, one is also at risk for developing diabetes. This shared risk, in turn, strengthens the ties of Chicago's intertribal community by binding together the citizens of many tribal nations as an ethnic enclave of Indigenous Americans.

While being at risk for developing diabetes is certainly not the most salient feature of Indigenous identity in Native Chicago, discussions of a shared biology do serve to strengthen ties in a community that is made up of individuals whose ancestors came from distant locations across North America. These discussions evoke a sense of community, while further distinguishing Native communities from settler communities by contrasting the purity of ancestral Native diets and bodies to the impurity of the settler diets.

Human knowledge is tentative; it is ephemeral; it is located in particular historic moments. In this chapter I described how diabetes is understood in contemporary Native Chicago. The ubiquity of the disease in the community influences local understandings of what the condition is and why people develop it. In defining diabetes, experiences with the biomedical model through human interaction and through media (like diabetes pamphlets distributed in social centers like the American Indian Center of Chicago) play a role, in addition to experiences of living with, caring for, and/or witnessing diabetes care in the community. Within these discussions, there is an underlying discourse of a shared evolutionary history that serves to strengthen the intertribal community bonds in the city.

In the next chapter I describe diabetes care in the community, demonstrating how members of this population are working together to care for the disease and how intertribal ties are strengthened through this shared work.

6

Care in the Context of Chronicity

On an unseasonably cool day in late July 2013, Regina, Roy, and I were plating the elder meal as an assembly line at the American Indian Center of Chicago. This Wednesday the smoky charred scent of burnt rice permeated the kitchen as we portioned out plates with a chicken taco, refried beans, rice carefully scooped from the top of the pan, and small condiment tubs of salsa and guacamole that we had portioned out earlier. As Regina was urging us to move faster to get the plates ready for the servers coming in and out, we stopped and exchanged glances of concern upon hearing an unexpected voice booming just outside the kitchen walls. Another volunteer poked her head outside the door to investigate the situation. She reported back that it was just Joshua making an announcement about the SoBe beverages that had been donated to the center. Joshua was telling his fellow lunch goers that they should not drink this product if they are diabetic, explaining that the nutrition label on the bottle was misleading. The twenty-ounce bottle contained 2.5 servings—meaning that if one person were to drink the entire bottle, they would consume a total of sixty-two grams of carbohydrates, and not the twenty-five listed on the nutrition panel. Many care providers encourage diabetic patients to consume meals containing between forty-five and sixty grams of carbohydrates per meal depending upon their care plan. Drinking this beverage in full would account for more than the recommend meal's worth of carbohydrates for any diabetic person.

Joshua's announcement to the lunch attendees represents one component of the diabetes care work being performed in Chicago's Native population. Care in this context is done within and across multiple spheres, from inside individual households to community-wide considerations. Because diabetes is a chronic condition that can result in serious and sometimes life-threatening complications if left uncontrolled—for instance amputation, blindness, and kidney and heart disease—mainstream physicians typically expect patients with this diagnosis to perform a set of daily tasks to mitigate the risk. These include testing blood glucose levels, counting and limiting the grams of carbohydrates in all consumed foods and beverages, exercising, examining feet for wounds, taking oral medications, and/or injecting shots of insulin.

This chapter explores care expectations and care practices in Native Chicago. In the first section, I look at expectations for care as described by biomedical providers in Chicago. I then explore local discourses from both patient and provider perspectives about factors that influence the performance of diabetes care work, describing how expectations of disease management differ between these caregivers. In the remainder of the chapter I focus on when, where, and how care work is performed, and by whom—investigating the direct and indirect acts of care being performed by men, women, and children in individual households and on a community-wide level. Ultimately, I argue that in this highly affected community care for diabetes goes far beyond individual self-care. Here, I extend studies of care by demonstrating how, in a community facing epidemic rates of disease, care is enmeshed in the everyday lives not just of those living with it but also of those in their lives. Members of Chicago's Native community incorporate not only diabetes care but awareness of other chronic condition needs into their lives, and this care is performed by individuals living with the disease, their family and friends, and at times the larger community.

This diabetes care work is one way in which ties in Chicago's inter-tribal community are strengthened.

Taking Control of Diabetes

People living with diabetes manage their blood glucose levels in order to prevent the development of secondary complications, which can be life-threatening. As described in earlier chapters, diabetes is a chronic condition characterized by elevated glucose levels in the blood stream due to insulin deficiency or insulin resistance. Over time, uncontrolled glucose levels can lead to the development of several complications, including heart disease, kidney disease and failure, amputation of toes, feet, legs and hands, and impaired vision or blindness. The tasks for managing diabetes vary from patient to patient, but they include some combination of testing blood glucose levels, counting and limiting the carbohydrates in all food and beverages consumed, taking oral medications and/or subcutaneous injections of insulin, and increasing physical activity. The majority of this care work is completed outside of the biomedical setting, by patients and family caregivers. The seeking of professional medical care is sporadic for some community members. While some people seek health care regularly, others either choose to or can only afford to go to a doctor only when absolutely necessary.

In Chicago, Natives have access to a variety of health-care options, including private and public health centers. Enrolled tribal citizens can receive free or very low-cost care from American Indian Health Service of Chicago. In cases where individuals do not have insurance, they can use this local resource and others, including Cook County Hospital; however, the cost of time to utilize some of these resources is high. Participants describe full days in the waiting room to get in for an appointment at Cook County Hospital, a health center southwest of the city's downtown that can take a long time to reach via public transportation from the northern side of the city, where many Chicago Natives reside. As described in chapter 1, due to rising housing costs brought about by gentrification, the majority of the city's Indigenous population now lives west of the Uptown neighborhood that was once the center of urban Indigenous life in Chicago. Yet, at the time of this research, American Indian Health Service of Chicago was located in Uptown. For this reason, several interviewees described the agency as being difficult to get to; additionally, it was difficult to schedule an appointment due to limited physician staffing onsite.[1] Furthermore, participants complained of the care they received there. Some interviewees thought the providers were judgmental, and some were uncomfortable with the quick pace of staff turnover. At the same time, many Chicago Natives do utilize American Indian Health Service of Chicago and describe it as a great benefit to the community because it allows them to access care at a relatively low cost. Lastly, some community members seek health care on their home reservations on annual or semiannual visits.

Biomedical providers working with the community describe focusing on developing individualized treatment plans that take individual lifestyles and needs into account. Janice, a thirty-year-old nurse of Ojibwe ancestry, explained her approach for working with diabetes patients:

> JANICE: Every person, I think I would say from my experience every patient is individualized and each patient care plan should be different because everybody's different. It's individually based because what we do here is that we do a referral from either the doctor or myself and refer the patient over to the, to the dietician, and she creates a meal plan for them. So we have anywhere from like a, I want to say a fifteen-hundred calorie diet to an eighteen-hundred calorie diet if I'm not mistaken. But it's, they're different, based on what their needs are, what their level of education is, and how their habits have been.

Non-Native nurse Leah Weitzel explained that while treatment plans are individualized, many diabetes care routines factor in some combination of the same lifestyle components:

LEAH: Well, healthy eating, however you want to do your carbohydrate, whether you want to literally count it or do the plate method, or whatever, but keeping that within the recommended guidelines. And a balanced diet, portion control—you can eat what you want but you have to watch when and how much you eat. And then regular, preferably daily, some sort of physical activity, but definitely several times a week and of moderate intensity. And then also stress management, I think it's important for both, because for it being a chronic disease and in order to practice the other healthy behaviors, a lot of times the stress has to be under control in the first place. And communication with family members and friends and whoever else may be involved so they understand what you need to do to practice those sort of healthy behaviors.

Leah did not mention medication but instead focused on the lifestyle changes individuals make to achieve diabetes control outside of the medical encounter. Biomedical providers recommend that people living with diabetes make significant lifestyle adjustments and perform acts of self-surveillance and discipline to achieve diabetes control. As Leah noted, providers do not anticipate that this care is entirely done by the patient alone, recognizing instead that it may also be supported through the efforts of family and friends.

"I Knew I Had It": Factors That Influence Care

Not all people with diabetes diagnoses make lifestyle adjustments or follow care plans in the manner suggested by their biomedical providers, for a variety of reasons. Local nurses express frustration with such cases. Violet, a non-Native volunteer nurse at the American Indian Center of Chicago, discussed how she worked with patients who have high blood glucose during the weekly health screenings at the center:

VIOLET: Well, I've gotten to know some of the people that work here. I usually ask them if they took their insulin this morning and if it's real high you know . . . we're supposed to follow up on it but some of these people have been diabetics for years so they know [in a characterized voice] "oh yeah I had I had ice cream last night or I had a big fudge sundae" or whatever they had or in the morning [in a characterized voice] "oh I had two donuts and I had coffee and this and that" so you know you try to tell them that you know maybe once in a while you can have a donut or half a donut but two donuts in the morning, I mean that's a bad start. Sugar goes up and then [in] a couple of hours it'll just drop.

Violet was concerned that not all patients understand the relationship between food intake and blood glucose readings, as indicated in her characterization of patient statements about eating ice cream and donuts without realizing the effect it might have on their blood glucose levels later in the day. Violet tried to educate those she encountered by talking with them about diet and offering diabetes pamphlets and magazines to refer to at home. An important point here is that while biomedical practitioners may hold expectations for patient self-care that are not feasible within this community, these practitioners sincerely care about the people they work with. Violet obtained these pamphlets from local contacts in Chicago's medical community on her own time to redistribute at the center. But she also got frustrated with patients who she thought just do not care, and with seeing her suggestions being disregarded by some individuals whom she genuinely aimed to provide care for.

During the period encompassed by my fieldwork, both the staff and volunteer nurses at the center kept mental lists of community members who they believed were not performing diabetes care tasks, and in meetings they would discuss these individuals and possible methods of promoting what they would describe as better diabetes care. In a June 2009 meeting, Violet and wellness director Mary discussed one community member who they knew was living with diabetes but opted to never have her blood glucose levels tested onsite during health screenings. Since this community member participated regularly in the blood pressure portion of the health screening, both Mary and Violet assumed that the woman was likely concerned that her glucose readings would be high and did not want to have it tested and recorded on site. In cases like this, wellness staff and volunteers discussed possible options for motiving diabetes care, including finding ways to lower costs of medications and testing supplies for use at home, or providing information about diet and nutrition in an approachable way.

Biomedical providers working with Chicago's Native community identify diagnosis avoidance and noncompliance with prescribed treatment as two significant challenges to diabetes care. Dacia, who has worked as a community health worker for over a decade, related why community members do not always seek biomedical care. In a conversation on intergenerational trauma I asked her to speak about the effects it can have on one's health:

> DACIA: Noncompliance . . . the patients that walk in our doors are patients who are oozing with an open wound. They're not coming in for preventative medicine. They come in because they are feeling so ill that they are you know, they are not able to operate. And they've waited. They've known there's been a symptom for so long, but they ignore it. And so everybody knows, like when we think of especially like diabetes, I want to say [the] community by and large knows the symptoms. It isn't that they don't, but so many times community members are like at the very, you know like in terms of finding out that they're, their sugars are out of whack, they've been out of whack for years. And they're just now walking in the door. You know and it's like their A1cs are at 10s, 11s, you know and it's like you know you're not even, they're not even finding out prediabetic or you know like something like that, they're finding out when it's already full-blown, like you've already done damage to your body kind of mode. And they still don't do anything about it. They still, they might take the medicine, just like, just like anybody. You have some kind of illness, you take your antibiotics 'til you're feeling better and you're like, oh I don't need it anymore. [forty-one-year-old Oneida community health worker]

Dacia used "full-blown" to refer to the development of diabetes in biomedical terms—the individual is no longer prediabetic but meets the diagnostic criteria of having diabetes. As a community health worker and an active community member, Dacia has seen the long-term ramifications that intergenerational trauma and depression have taken on Chicago Natives.

I realized the gravity of the situation described by Dacia in the course of another interview, with Roy. Roy and I had worked together on various events at the center over the year before our interview. His mother has diabetes, and he has expressed concern that he is likely to develop the disease in the future. Still, Roy explained that he was not ready to find out his status vis à vis diabetes at that point in his life:

MEG: Do you ever get screened for it?

ROY: No.

MEG: Have you thought about?

ROY: I've thought about but then thinking about it's like if you really want to know it's like going to change your whole life. And right now I don't want that to change. [thirty-five-year-old Oglala Sioux/Navajo man with diabetic family members]

Roy's ambivalence about learning whether he has diabetes serves here as an example of Dacia's description of diabetes in the community. Roy knew about diabetes, its symptoms, its complications, and the risk factors he has for developing it. In the years since that interview, he has actively been trying to lose weight through exercise and diet. While he is making lifestyle changes that could prevent the development of diabetes, he is still not at a point in his life where he would like to know if he has already developed it.

Clinicians and nonclinicians alike use the language of denial to describe this pattern. However, in Roy's case, he did not express any concern about current symptoms. Sylvia's experience more clearly exemplifies Dacia's description of an individual knowing that they are displaying trademark diabetes symptoms but not immediately seeking diagnosis. In our interview, Sylvia explained that she knew for a while that she was displaying the trademark diabetes symptoms but could not bring herself to see a doctor for some time:

> SYLVIA: I've been feeling like this for about a couple months, I know something's wrong with me but I just I hated to face it. Like I denied it that I had it. But I really knew I had it but, I just say no I don't have it. [sixty-nine-year-old Chippewa woman]

Sylvia went on to explain that she only sought diagnosis after being prompted by Laura at the American Indian Center's wellness program to follow up on the health screening performed at the center. Multiple interviewees described an experience like Sylvia's, where they were motivated to seek diagnosis and care for diabetes by the program, underscoring how vital informal wellness programs are for to supporting community health.

While biomedical providers and some community members describe some diabetics in the community as not caring for their diabetes, people living with the condition have alternate understandings of their level of disease management. Both biomedical providers and community members speak of diabetes care in terms of control. Medical anthropologists also describe how experiences of health and illness are discussed in terms of patient control over identity. Gay Becker describes how diagnosis with a chronic condition can cause someone to feel a loss of control for a period of time. The acute nature of diagnosis, Becker explains, is replaced as chronicity sets in and the patient reorients themselves, adjusting their life to the condition with which they have been diagnosed, thereby regaining control.[2] Dorothy Broom and Andrea Whittaker point out that in the case of diabetes discourses in Australia, patients speak about diabetes in moralizing terms of control. As they argue, people negotiate their patient identity through explaining their reduced levels of control by evoking the image of children, effectively lowering their agentive abilities when describing themselves as not following their diabetes care routine.[3] Individual experiences of health and disease are articulated using the language of control of individual bodies and choices. Self-surveillance is the cornerstone of contemporary diabetes care and other chronic condition care as prescribed by mainstream physicians. But the reality of completing this type of care is far more complicated, particularly in a case like diabetes, where the symptoms can be ignored while the patient tends to more pressing life matters.

Control is also a central topic in discussions of diabetes care in Native Chicago, as individuals seek to identify themselves and their ability to perform certain types of care acts on their own terms. There is a range of explanations for why individuals do not perform care tasks in the way suggested by biomedical providers. The most common include the high financial costs of eating healthier diets and obtaining medical supplies, the difficulty in accessing fresh foods in contrast to the ease of picking up processed food items that tend to have higher carbohydrate counts, and the time constraints of diabetes care in the city. Often diabetics describe being asymptomatic, even though they have high blood glucose readings. Carmen explained that she depends upon technology to care for diabetes:

CARMEN: I've never been able to tell when it was high . . . I can't feel no symptoms . . . So the only thing that will work with that then is to take your count. [sixty-nine-year-old Oneida woman living with diabetes]

Many people share Carmen's experience of not feeling a difference between what are defined as normal and high blood glucose levels. Normal blood glucose ranges are determined individually by biomedical providers. Participants defined their normal ranges to vary between 65 and 120 mg/dL for before meals, and below 180 mg/dL after meals. While high glucose levels are less often recognized, the experience of low blood glucose levels is described as being felt in dramatic ways—sweating, feeling overheated, shaking, feeling dizzy, and being unable to concentrate. These experiences were described as occurring rarely, but were very memorable to those who went through them.

One of the largest burdens faced by people living with diabetes in the community is the high cost of diabetes care. These costs are closely tied to at-home care technology involving blood glucose testing devices. The test strips for these devices are expensive. The price of a single blood glucose test strip ranges from $0.20 to $1.60, and physicians expect diabetics to test their glucose levels between two and six times daily. In addition to the high cost of testing supplies are the high costs of pharmaceuticals for diabetes treatment and of eating a healthy diet. While some interviewees described fully comprehending the suggested diet that they should follow living with diabetes, they found that meeting these requirements was outside their reach.

> JOAN: Well I see her [the dietician] but then the stuff she tells you are like impossible. I tell her sometimes when you're on a fixed income it's impossible to buy what you're supposed to have. [forty-nine-year-old Potawatomi/Puerto Rican woman living with diabetes]

Financial burdens are high in chronic condition care and this burden affects care practices. As noted in an earlier chapter, more than 20 percent of participants in the 2015 survey I conducted were living below the national poverty line, and at that time 37 percent reported that they did not have health-care coverage of any kind. There is a danger in placing blame on patients for not performing care activities without first understanding the larger context in which care is or is not being done.

When diabetes patients do not feel ill and cannot afford blood glucose testing machines and supplies, their diabetes management is done on their own terms. Sylvia described that though she cannot afford the test strips to measure her blood glucose levels as frequently as her doctor recommends, she takes advantage of all opportunities provided to her to test her levels for free, including the health screenings at the center and at local pharmacies:

> SYLVIA: They check it over here [the center], or sometimes I go to that store where they got the machine, I check it there . . . When I'm walking by CVS, I'm, oh I'll check my blood sugars. I'm going to go check my blood sugars.

From the point of view of mainstream health-care providers, Sylvia may be seen as not caring for her diabetes; however, from her own point of view, she is doing the best she can in her circumstances.

While some diabetics in Native Chicago describe themselves as striving to do the best they can, others describe a conscious choice to not follow biomedical recommendations for care. This choice is at times articulated in terms of performing a Native identity. Gerard went for nearly a decade of his life without taking medication for diabetes after being diagnosed. In our interview, Gerard related his story, beginning with his borderline diagnosis in the 1990s and ending with his decision in the late fall of 2012 to begin taking prescription medications:

GERARD: When I found out I was borderline and they said I could control with weight and diet and all that stuff, I was like, okay, it wasn't a big deal to me. So when it came time for my next appointment, it didn't get any, it didn't decline any. It didn't really advance. I was still kind of like in the same area, so they started talking about medication and that's what kind of, I just don't like, I've never taken drugs, that's kind of my claim to fame, I've never taken any kind of drug, you know like prescribed sure for whatever, but nothing illegal. So when they started talking about medication, it kind of freaked me out. I had a negative vibe to it and I just, so from that point on, they're like if you, your next visit if you're the same or advance, they go, you're going to be taking medication.

And so from that point on, I didn't go to the doctor because I knew in my heart that I wasn't doing anything to, to fix the situation. Eventually I thought ah, it'll go away. I mean I really thought that . . . I stopped doing the pin pricking to see my blood count, I stopped doing that. I just stopped everything and just kind of lived life and eating unhealthy, not really exercising, I was gaining a lot of weight, so I knew that, and then of course, I understood the symptoms of diabetes, like frequent urination and fatigue and those two you know, and then, and then it was the urination that I knew that my blood was high. But yeah, you know I just didn't do anything about it ... I was borderline [in] '91, never really professionally, nobody ever told me I was diabetic up until maybe six or seven years ago but then I finally started taking oral medication as of October of last year [2012] ... Yes, and I probably trimmed a lot of years off my life, but I don't know. But I think that's, I think that's how I feel in my heart is that I lessened my lifetime (laughs). I laugh about it maybe it's just a nervous laugh, but yeah. [forty-four-year-old Choctaw/Navajo man living with diabetes]

Acutely aware of the symptoms and possible complications, Gerard described knowing that by not caring for diabetes at the beginning he was trimming years off his life. Later in our conversation, Gerard shared:

GERARD: Every time my diabetes comes into question, people are like, people who know my family are like, didn't [your] grandfather pass away because of complications from diabetes? I'm like yes. They're like, and then they would say don't you know people who get their arms or feet amputated? And I'm like yes, I know people like that. They're like, why don't you learn from that. And I was like I don't know. I'm very aware of it, I know the complications, I know that you could go blind, [have a] heart attack, stroke, I know all that can happen, but why doesn't it happen, why doesn't it help me. I don't know, maybe it is a mental thing ... I do think the Creator has, and this is where people just like roll their eyes at me or just think I'm being silly, but I do believe Creator does have a path in mind for me ... I'm not saying I should not do anything about my diabetes. Obviously, I am, because I started taking the medication, but if it so happens I get heart failure because of diabetes, then I think that was the path that was given to me. So, I am at a point in my life where I'm like yeah, Western medicine is going to help, it's going to help. I've come to that conclusion. And it was recent, within the last five years. So why didn't I take medication five years ago when I had that revelation or epiphany, I don't know, I just felt for some reason last October.

It was in the early 1990s that Gerard was first diagnosed as a borderline diabetic and he chose at that time to not follow up with future visits. In his account, Gerard focuses on his choice to not care for diabetes in the way biomedicine recommends, first attributing his choice of not taking medications as "silliness" and youth, and later relating this to his Native identity and relationship with Creator and Creator's path for him, which he later in life felt did not preclude him from taking diabetes medications.

The choice to not use Western medicine or take pills was described as being related to a distinctly Native behavior in other instances in this community as well. Lyle, a forty-seven-year-old Menominee/Ho-Chunk man, described how his mother would check her blood glucose, but was "hard-headed"—a trait he linked with being Native in several contexts in our interview—in terms of her diabetes care needs:

> LYLE: She's having some diabetic issues in regard to amputation issues, but she's hard-headed and she doesn't want that kind of thing to happen and she'd rather just live with it and whatever, you know, because of the Native American thing, but she lives in Wisconsin right now, so she's kind of undecided about that, so she has some cancer issues too.
>
> MEG: Can I ask what you meant by the Native American thing?
>
> LYLE: Just the belief system that she, yeah, she doesn't want, she's not going to let anybody cut anything off her body that shouldn't be cut off.

Explanations for care practices that do not meet biomedical recommendations incorporate Native identity into the narrative. Both Gerard and Lyle describe rejecting and avoiding Western medical intervention as a Native characteristic. Some Natives distrust the biomedical community, a distrust based upon histories of maltreatment in health-care services and health research.[4] Because of these histories, urban Indigenous Americans describe being apprehensive of biomedical research and health care. While both Native and non-

Native nondiabetics may define the actions of people like Gerard as not taking care of their diabetes, people living with diabetes have alternate understandings of their level of disease management that is built upon their capabilities for caring for the disease in their current circumstances; they also define their care in relation to their identity as an individual, as a patient, and as a person of Indigenous ancestry.

Depression and stress are two additional factors that play a role in diabetes care practices in the community. While the experience of living with diabetes often include life burdens brought on by the disease, for instance, financial hardship, depression, increased stress, and physical limitations, 72.5 percent of those living with diabetes interviewed for this research were also caring for additional illnesses. These include high blood pressure, high cholesterol, arthritis, mobility limitations, cancer, depression, irritable bowel syndrome, bipolar disorder, and HIV. The high occurrence of comorbidities in this population is of importance. As noted earlier, not all people living with diabetes notice the symptoms of the disease. In early cases of diabetes, symptoms may not hinder day-to-day life, while other more pressing health and life concerns require immediate attention and action. Health-care providers say that diabetes is a manageable disease, but it is one that takes time, patience, and practice. Community health worker Dacia believed that depression inhibits care practices:

> DACIA: I was working with her [a diabetic patient], trying to make sure at the time she was on insulin, and you know I'm always asking her, how are your feet doing and how is everything going, and going through everything, the long list. Oh, you know I noticed there was something on the bottom of my other foot. What's on the, what's going on? She's like I don't know, it's kind of a, an open sore. Not what you want to hear, right? And then it's like well, I know you were telling me last week you had a podiatrist appointment, when is that appointment? (sigh) I don't know. That's in my other purse. And because this is a home visit and we're sitting there staring at each other, could we, could we find out when that is?

Oh I don't know. I'm physically right here. Right here at your disposal. You can tell me where the purse is, I can go get it for you. You could help yourself to it. All that I want it for is so I have an idea of when that appointment is so I can make sure that I'm calling you, reminding you that you have this appointment, you need to go in and if you're not going in, we need to be calling immediately, getting you into the doctor because you already lost one toe. I don't know, I'm not a medical professional to understand the whatever's this wound looks like. But I do know enough to know that if it's an open wound, you need to be in there. 'Cause your blood sugar is too high. Oh, can I just call you back for that information. It's like depression to the ninth degree, right. It's like anything that's preventing you from keeping yourself healthy from like that downward.

Diabetes, from Dacia's viewpoint, can be worsened if one is dealing with depression and intergenerational trauma. Though members of Chicago's Native community do not often link intergenerational trauma to diabetes development, they do associate the effects of the trauma to depression and to issues of "noncompliance," in Dacia's terms. Several diabetes patients confirmed Dacia's explanation, elaborating on how depression hinders care work from time to time, while others also described diabetes as a contributing factor to their depression and other mental health concerns.

Family Motivating Care

While these issues challenging care in the community are significant concerns, care work is being performed in direct and indirect ways. Family members of all generations influence care practices performed by patients. While Gerard explained that he had witnessed family and friends succumb to diabetes complications, he for a time was unmoved by these experiences to perform certain care acts, like taking medications. Others in similar circumstances had the opposite reaction. Kenneth, a twenty-year-old Cherokee/ white man, was motivated to care for his diabetes by witnessing his uncle's complications from the disease:

KENNETH: My uncle, that's the one that I had seen went blind. He's the one that influenced me to keep on like checking my stuff a lot, more than I should, and keep an eye on track so that I don't end up like he did.

While Kenneth is motivated to avoid the complications his uncle suffered from, others see younger generations as motivating care. Doris, a forty-seven-year-old Potawatomi/Puerto Rican woman, told me she looks forward to being there for her family in the future:

DORIS: What motivates me is my grandkids, you know to be there for them, to take care of them, 'cause like I said, they're, one's autistic and it's you know nobody really wants to take care of an autistic kid unless you have to, and so I'm trying really hard to make sure that I can be here longer to help with that one, I know I've been bad in the past and laid up in the hospital, but this time I'm trying to just straighten it all out.

Doris and others explained that they perform diabetes care not for themselves but with their family in mind. According to a study conducted by Laura Heinemann, people on the wait list for an organ transplant often explain that they do not want the organ for themselves, but to be around to support others in their lives.[5] This same reason is cited in Native Chicago, where people strive to care for diabetes to fulfill personal and familial obligations and responsibilities.

Gender and Care

Both men and women in Chicago's Native community are involved in the day-to-day care of diabetes. In interviews with participants living with the disease, we discussed their daily care routine and whether they receive help from others. Women are caring for their diabetes on their own more often than men: 92 percent of diabetic women (twenty-three of twenty-five interviewed) stated that they did not have another person helping them care for diabetes, while 53.3 percent of male diabetics (eight of fifteen interviewed) stated that they did not receive help. For both the male and female diabetics I spoke with at the time, the majority saw themselves as the only person involved in their daily care for the disease.

In interviews with family members of diabetics, more women than men described themselves as being involved in diabetes care: 70.6 percent of women (twelve of seventeen interviewed) and 61.5 percent of men (eight of thirteen interviewed) said they were involved in the care of family members with diabetes. They described their care work as including shopping, cooking, doing research, changing their own eating habits, sympathizing, attending medical appointments, administering insulin injections, and running errands with patients; 23.5 percent of women (four of seventeen interviewed) and 46.2 percent of men (six of thirteen interviewed) stated that they were not involved in the day-to-day care of diabetes for family members. The four women and three of the six men who said they were not involved explained their noninvolvement as due to living too far away from the family member to participate in care. The three remaining men simply stated that they were just not involved.

In Chicago's Native community, female diabetics often prioritize care for their families over care for themselves. Based on our conversations, it seems for many of these women, the care for diabetes may not be as pressing of a concern as some family matters. In one of our discussions, Tammy, a sixty-eight-year-old Oneida woman, described how she was once able to control her diabetes through diet alone, but because of her family's fixed income, she and her husband, who had other health concerns, could not always afford to eat separate meals:

> TAMMY: Of course to eat a certain kind of food and to fix it a certain kind of way and everything else like this and that. We didn't have that kind of money. We were both on fixed incomes. We were both on disability, so I mean we couldn't just go out and get what just what I had to eat and then say get him what he wanted to eat. It was just too expensive.

In a later interview, Tammy expanded further on how she managed her care in the household as her husband's health deteriorated:

TAMMY: Because of taking my husband here, bringing him home, taking him there the next day, you know, so I never had time to have a balanced meal. I'd make sure when we got home, my husband was hungry, I'd fix him something and then I'd just go ahead and [eat] anything that was fixable, or just throw together a sandwich in the fridge. Well that's what I would fix, you know for myself. [It] was really rough at that time, and so I didn't take, I wasn't taking my medicine for one thing because I knew that, well I was supposed to eat meals, then take my medicine.

In Tammy's description, she was responsible for caring for the family and preparing foods for the family to consume. Her health took a secondary place as she forewent her own health needs to care for her husband's— prioritizing his dietary concerns and care needs over her own.

Almeda saw this as a continuing problem today among her tribe on the Choctaw reservation. She believed that while many diabetic men will go without caring for their diabetes, women will seek to monitor and care for the disease but will be prevented from eating properly by their household responsibilities to their families:

ALMEDA: But I think the reason why they cause them so much problem to stick to their diet is there, see they have some children, they have children and a husband and they have to cook for them. If she cooks a diabetic way, they not going to eat. They going to be complaining. And then by the time that you get through cooking for them, you're too tired to cook for yourself. [seventy-seven-year-old Choctaw woman living with diabetes]

Men in the community also prioritize the health of a spouse over their own. Miguel, a sixty-year-old diabetic Menominee man, describes how he put off his own health needs in order to care for his wife:

MIGUEL: I was too involved with my wife being home, taking her home for hospice, so I just left all my, I left all my medical stuff off to the side until I got everything situated and I went back in 2010 and started getting taken care of myself.

Miguel suffered a heart attack at the hospital while staying with his wife, who was there for her own health concerns. It was during this event that he learned that he had diabetes. As he explains, he focused his attention at the time on his ailing wife and did not return to the doctor for his heart condition or his diabetes until several years later, after his wife passed.

Childcare and work obligations can also interfere with individual care routines. Carmen described how she focused more on caring for her grandchildren than on managing her diabetes. Having several young children to get off to school each morning and a demanding job as the social services director at a local community center, Carmen had little time for adhering to regimented orders in caring for a disease she does not feel:

> CARMEN: I don't eat regular like I should I try to, but it's so hard when you gotta go to work and this and that and you just don't have time . . . I usually forget to take my medicine . . . So usually when they come, the American Indian Health comes on Wednesdays . . . it [her blood glucose level] is usually pretty high. It's in the two hundreds you know. [sixty-nine-year-old Oneida woman living with diabetes]

According to Carmen, her doctors had been "getting on her case" for not monitoring her diabetes as they had instructed her. However, as evident in Carmen's statements, balancing time between work, family, and personal care was difficult, and when she did not feel physically ill from diabetes, she did not prioritize its care over other pressing family and work concerns.

For both male and female diabetics, their own health may take a backseat to other household concerns. They prioritize their responsibilities as spouses, parents, grandparents, and employees over that of caring for diabetes. It is important to note here that the majority of the diabetics I spoke with do not always feel physically ill when their blood sugar is higher than what doctors describe as normal—so the urgency of caring for diabetes may not be immediately felt, while family care or work responsibilities may be a more pressing concern. For both male and female diabetics, the majority of each group describe themselves as the sole caregiver for their diabetes management. However, women are more often without additional assistance than are men. Women also more frequently describe their prioritization of household work and family needs over diabetes care, while both men and women equally describe prioritizing their employment obligations over care. Rebecca Seligman and colleagues describe a similar situation in Mexican American diabetes care in Chicago, where family care can take priority over diabetes management.[6]

Children Providing Care

Because diabetes is so prevalent in Chicago's Native population, children are aware of the disease at a young age, often first learning of the disease through observing and witnessing the care routines of adult family members. In many instances, children participate in care work. Kevin is a thirty-two-year-old Ojibwe man who grew up in a family surrounded by diabetes. For Kevin, giving his mother injections of insulin was part of his childhood and something that he continued to do in adulthood:

> KEVIN: Basically just like whenever she needs to get shot up, you know, that's what I do. She puts, she fills it, whatever amount she needs in it, then she pinches herself and I got to shoot it. I've been doing it since I been a kid. That's just something I grew up [with] naturally.

As Kevin explained in our conversation, he lives with his mother and returns home throughout the day to administer his mother's insulin. This is not unusual, as children have been seen to incorporate themselves into the care work of family in the context of epidemics across the globe. Jean Hunleth's discussion of tuberculosis treatment in Zambia focuses on the role that children play in ensuring parent tuberculosis patients adhere to their medical treatment regimens. In the context of the tuberculosis and HIV epidemic in Zambia, these children perform care practices to protect the future of their childhood by helping their parent survive.[7] In Chicago, care provided by younger generations involves the administering of medications, in addition to cooking and providing reminders for care. Aria, a thirty-four-year-old Assiniboine woman, described how her children monitor her eating:

> ARIA: The kids are pretty good about it. They're the worst when they catch me eating something I shouldn't be ... Mom, the doctor said you're not supposed to have that. Mom, you're going to have to give yourself insulin. Mom!

Aria's children, like Kevin, learned to participate in diabetes care in early in life. This early childhood involvement can transition into adult care work as Chicago Natives age.

Tiffany, now a thirty-nine-year-old Seneca woman, described how in her teens she researched information on diabetes so that she could help take care of her grandfather when she lived with him on the reservation during summers:

> TIFFANY: I talked to the nurse. We have a community building on our reservation and it has a clinic inside, so I went in there and I asked her, you know what is diabetes, what is that stuff, you know. And she's like oh, and gave me all kinds of books and pamphlets and everything. So I did my own research, and I'm like, oh okay. I knew what he could have and what he couldn't have, so. And then I had to start cooking for him too, because that's when I knew he wasn't supposed to have some of the things that he was having, you know.

Tiffany translated this diabetes care learned on the reservation to her Chicago home a decade later when her father was diagnosed with diabetes. Now in her late thirties, Tiffany is utilizing this knowledge again to prevent her eleven-year-old daughter, who was diagnosed as being borderline diabetic, from fully developing the condition.

Children growing up in Chicago's Native community become aware of diabetes at a young age and some take on the role of caregiver for their family members. The knowledge of diabetes and its care needs increases with age and many children who first observe and participate in diabetes care in childhood continue to do so as adults, both within families and within the larger community.

Living with Diabetics

In the context of this epidemic there are many households where there is more than one diabetic living in the home. In these instances, diabetes patients receive additional assistance from their fellow diabetics in both direct and indirect ways. In Helena's home, both she and her husband were diabetic. Before her husband passed, they would take turns testing the other's blood glucose levels—a task both of them disliked:

> HELENA: You do mine [blood glucose test] today and I'll do yours tomorrow. So we worked out a little game plan to how to deal with it because they tell you, well, you got to do this and you got to do that. Well, yeah, but there's a way to deal with it. [sixty-eight-year-old Apache woman living with diabetes]

Though Helena and her husband were testing their blood glucose levels less frequently than what was recommended by their physicians, they were doing some testing at home through the assistance of one another. Diabetics living with other diabetes patients describe other forms of direct care they exchange, including shopping for diabetes-friendly foods, cooking low-carbohydrate and low-fat meals to share, and walking together for exercise. Not all care assistance, however, is performed through direct actions. Diabetics living with other diabetics describe receiving a great deal of help in the household by just seeing a sibling or a spouse in their own diabetes care routine. For instance, seeing a glucometer or medications in a central area of the home serves as a reminder for individuals to take medication and test blood glucose levels.

While patients help one another, they also receive both direct and indirect forms of assistance from nondiabetics both living with them and otherwise. In an interview, Steven described his wife as a "watch dog" who reminds him what he can and cannot have to eat. In an interview with his wife, Susan, she explained how her husband's having the disease has not only changed his lifestyle but has altered their life together:

> SUSAN: We don't eat out. All our meals, most of the meals are prepared at home. If we do eat out it's off a light menu. [fifty-eight-year-old Seneca woman with diabetic family members]

Throughout our conversation Susan emphasized that the changes brought on by her husband's diabetes affected both of them by using the pronoun "we"—in describing trips to doctor's appointments and changes to the household diet. Susan's use of this plural first-person pronoun highlights her view that her husband's diagnosis was not one that just affected his life, but one that has altered their life together, so much so that she too orders off of a light menu when they go out to eat. Julie Livingston describes in her work on a cancer oncology ward in Botswana that cancer is not something that happens to a person, but something that occurs between people.[8] Livingston's suggestion is provocative for thinking about all types of human care, because it calls attention to the nature of illness and how individuals often experience it in multiple spheres, sharing the care experience with medical providers, family, friends, and support networks. Though the majority of both male and female diabetes patients in Chicago's Native community do not always describe the assistance they receive from others as care, work that thoughtfully takes diabetes needs and care into account is being performed in both direct and indirect ways. This care work, in a sense, is hidden.[9]

The meaning of care is shaped and defined by the context in which it is being performed. Care has to be understood in terms of local historic, economic, social, cultural, and political contexts. It can take on many forms, from direct actions of administering medications to indirect forms of support, such as eating similar meals to reduce feelings of difference. In her work on the logic of care and the logic of choice, Annemarie Mol describes how care is an open-ended process in which a care team is involved in the constant negotiation between technologies, knowledge, and local bodies.

Central to Mol's argument is that care is based in relationships—in her example of diabetes in a Dutch hospital, care is created in the relationship and engagements of patients, medical providers, and medical technologies.[10] In Duana Fullwiley's study of sickle cell in Senegal, she found what she defines as therapeutic economies—contexts in which sickle cell patients expand kin networks in the space of sickle cell patient groups where a sense of normalcy is developed among those sharing the disease.[11] In her study of diabetes care practices among Turkish women in Germany, Cornelia Guell describes how a diagnosis with diabetes affects family and social life. She shows that the women mitigate the effect of diabetes in these spheres by creating ways to take care of their diabetes while participating in social norms, for instance, clearing their plate after eating and returning to the table to socialize without the risk of refilling their plate.[12] Caring for chronic conditions, then, is often woven into social worlds. In Native Chicago, men and women participate in visible and hidden care work.

In a community facing epidemic rates of disease, care—as thoughtful actions with diabetes treatment in mind—is enmeshed in the everyday lives of not just those living with the disease but also of those in and across their communities. Members of Chicago's Native community incorporate care for diabetes and other chronic conditions into their lives, not only for diabetics but also for their family, friends, and even the larger community. Care in this context involves a wide range of activities: conducting research, attending appointments, shopping, cooking, administering medications, doing exercise, eating diabetes diets when not diabetic, reminding patients about foods, watching for signs of hyperglycemia in others, providing education and advice, and considering diet needs for larger community events. Through care work, ties binding members of Chicago's Native community are strengthened.

While it is easier to provide care for diabetes patients if one is living with them, living a distance from family members does not preclude one from being involved in diabetes care. Susan described how she calls her son living on a reservation in New York State to give him information that she has learned about diabetes management. Holly described how she helped her parents by picking up grocery items for them. After years of seeing her parents reject the sugar-free items she would purchase, she began to disguise these so that they would get the cookies they desired, but ones that were safer in her view for them to consume:

> HOLLY: I would look for you know anything diabetic friendly, sugar free, and I'd peel labels off, you know like I said, or I'd hide them or something so that they didn't know it was that way. 'Cause I knew if they saw the label, they wouldn't eat it. So I would do that. [forty-four-year-old Apache/Sioux woman with diabetic family members]

Some of the care that is provided is indirect as well. For many of the nondiabetic caregivers I spoke with, living with diabetics has led to the development of great sympathy for the struggles their family and friends face in dealing with the condition. Maintaining a diet low in fat and low in carbohydrates is what most diabetics I spoke with struggle with; each diabetic I spoke with had a favorite food or meal from their pre-diabetes life that they missed the most—ranging from frybread to Chicago dogs with a side of french fries. Nondiabetic caregivers describe how they sympathize with this difficulty, and how they participate in the diabetic lifestyle by eating the same foods as their diabetic family members in order to reduce any level of difference that the latter may feel due to their diabetes. Virginia described how during family functions there would be a wide spread of food that her father's diabetes restricted him from eating. Virginia explained:

> VIRGINIA: You could see it in his eyes but he couldn't have it . . . When I would see my dad eat, I would see a small portion of salad . . . And you would see him looking at other people's plates, and I knew what he was going through, so I didn't have steaks, or corn on the cob with butter on it, I didn't have soda. I used to eat kind of similar to what he had, so he wouldn't feel so bad. [thirty-one-year-old Navajo woman with diabetic family members]

Virginia spoke with a trembling voice of her witnessing her father's experience, expressing the degree to which she felt and shared her father's struggles with diabetes care. As Virginia explained throughout our interview, she strove to make her father feel less different, in hopes of encouraging him to eat a healthier diet to care for the condition.

Friends also provide support, knowing what diabetes can do to a person when left uncontrolled. Vincent, a fifty-five-year-old Seneca man, described how he chose to eat the same meals as his diabetic friend so that she would be less tempted to have the higher fat and higher carbohydrate meals.

> VINCENT: Whenever I was around Lois, I wouldn't eat things that I knew she couldn't eat, so I wouldn't eat them. She'd say I'm going to have a salad and this and I say, oh I'll have that too. You know that wasn't eating that greasy cheeseburger or fried chicken, I was just eating whatever she ate too. And she'd always tell me, no you eat something good. I said no that's alright with me.

Diabetes patients describe how this type of support is helpful for them, so that they do not feel a difference between their own actions and those of others. In Chicago's Native community, nondiabetics are involved in diabetes care in both direct and indirect ways—from Kevin administering insulin injections for his mother to Virginia and Vincent eating similar meals as their diabetic family and friends to support eating what is often viewed as less desirable food options.

Community Considerations of Diabetes Care

Diabetes care is not only carried out within the interpersonal relationships of family and friends; in Native Chicago, it is also considered on a communal level. For the winter holidays of 2013, Rebecca made more than sixty loaves of banana bread to share as a gift to elders at the American Indian Center. As she gave them to volunteers to help her distribute the bread at the senior lunch, she explained that half of the loaves were made with sugar and the other half were made with the low carbohydrate sweetener Splenda, intended for those who had diabetes. Members of Chicago's Native population are acutely aware of the prevalence of diabetes in the community and their actions are influenced and shaped by this knowledge. In Joshua's announcement to the senior lunch crowd, his warning was not intended for one friend or family member, but was meant for the wider community to hear and consider. Indigenous Americans in Chicago incorporate a concern for diabetes care for the community into their routines.

While individuals are shaping their actions with diabetes care in mind, community events are another space where diabetes care is considered. In an interview, Lois contrasted going out to eat at an event or restaurant outside the Native community with events held within Native society:

> LOIS: When you go places, I mean I went to a luncheon. It was like a diabetic nightmare. You know, every, the whole table's set up with nothing but sweets. You know, it's a luncheon, it's an honor, it's a birthday party for someone. Being a diabetic, it's like whoa, I'm not supposed to eat *any* of this. But I think people haven't adjusted to our diabetes yet and it should be more food out there. Restaurants should carry more food. I think if people would even get a restaurant where they have sugar-free food, I think it would do a great business. [fifty-eight-year-old Ojibwe woman living with diabetes]

Moments later Lois contrasted the food at these events with those held within the Native community:

> LOIS: They make vegetables and yeah, we can eat if we want to. You know there's a big selection of food, so you can adjust it to your [diet].

Staff and volunteers prepare a great number of meals and feasts within the kitchen of the American Indian Center each year, from the weekly senior luncheons to holiday events, town hall meetings, and community ceremonies. I observed during my time in this kitchen a significant transition from 2007, when it employed both a dietician and a chef, to 2016, when staff members from unrelated departments had taken up the reins to ensure that seniors had a weekly meal at which to socialize. Both before and after this transition, I noted that most of the meals are made with what the center can afford through its purchases from the Greater Chicago Food Depository and with what they can get for free from the depository. As discussed in the previous chapter, community health workers are concerned with the portion sizes of meals during community events, particularly large celebrations and holidays. As Lois notes, however, the availability of vegetables and other diabetic friendly food options at these events demonstrates an awareness of diabetes care needs in the community.

Today the staff and regular meal volunteers take not only diabetes into account when preparing meals but also high cholesterol, high blood pressure, dental concerns, and arthritis—rinsing off canned fruits and vegetables to reduce the amounts of sugar and sodium served to lunch attendees or peeling the skin off of fresh oranges served for dessert to cut back on food preparation labor for lunch goers with arthritis-swollen fingers. Helen, a twenty-two-year-old Arikara/Omaha/Odawa woman, and at the time of this interview staff cook at the center, explained her considerations for purchasing and preparing food for the senior meals:

> HELEN: I don't really like buying desserts. I usually forget about it and we pull out cans from back. No desserts, well I try to get them sugar free, if I, if I can get it from the food depository sugar free then I'll like load up on them ... I try giving them fresh fruit if, like if I know I have the time to stand there and cut it up, then I did it or someone to help. I like getting fresh fruit though, but also I'm trying, I try cooking with no salt. Yeah, none of the stuff I make I add salt to it. Most of the seasonings I have in the kitchen are salt free.

The American Indian Center hosted its first senior lunch at its new site on Ainslie Avenue in April of 2019. At this catered meal prepared by two Indigenous women, the health needs of the community were clearly in mind. The main course included low sodium meatloaf, mashed potatoes, and a three-sisters inspired veggie dish of corn, green beans, and squash. Dessert was a mixed wild berry crisp and whipped cream, both sweetened with the low carbohydrate sweetener Splenda. In Chicago's Native population, there is a heightened awareness at the community level of the health of its members. Community organizers consider these factors when organizing and preparing for gatherings, while individuals likewise think of the health of the larger population. Chicago's intertribal community is strengthened through the shared care work taken on by its members.

Care encompasses many things, from picking up pamphlets during one's personal time to share with community members, to eating diabetes-friendly meals with family and friends, and to drawing attention to the misleading nature of a food nutrition label. Diabetes care is thought about and performed on multiple levels in Chicago's Indigenous community. While diabetes patients may not immediately identify the work of their family members, friends, and community members as care, the work that is being done thoughtfully incorporates the needs and well-being of diabetics. Because there are high rates of the disease, children learn about it at a young age through first observing adult diabetes care and by later researching and becoming actively involved in care routines. Diabetes in the community is so common that there are many households with multiple diabetics within the home, creating a setting where they directly and indirectly participate in each other's care—from visual reminders to performing blood glucose tests. Care is further considered at the community level—where event organizers take diabetes into consideration (along with other community health needs) as they plan and prepare meals.

Chicago's Native community is strengthened through some of this care work. In the face of an epidemic characterized by chronicity, care for disease is woven into the everyday lives of community members. In this context, there is a heightened awareness beginning in childhood about diabetes and its detrimental effects on family and community members. Today members of Chicago's Native population are thinking about and acting upon community-wide health concerns—developing more varied diets for events, organizing and hosting the first 5K run event for the sixty-first annual American Indian Center Powwow held in September of 2014, hosting a group weight loss challenge inspired by the television series *The Biggest Loser*, and planting, tending, and monitoring Native gardens with traditional plants around the Chicago area. The care for this disease that so greatly affects Chicago's Native population is done within individual households and across multiple spheres of community life.

Conclusion

Rosanna and I were wrapping up our interview on her role as a diabetes caregiver when I asked what she would like to see for the future. Rosanna has observed and participated in her mother's care for diabetes throughout her adolescent and early adult life. Her response highlights the ways in which Chicago's intertribal Indigenous community comes together to address not only diabetes but improving community well-being more broadly:

ROSANNA: We don't really talk about it, like we're, we're going to prevent diabetes or [be] diabetes free. I think what's starting to take shape, or what has been taking shape for, at least as far as I know at least a decade, has been harvesting our own foods around our own area. And there have been like physical activity events here and there, and I think people are constantly trying those things out you know . . . Indian Health just hosted a weight loss challenge . . . I'd like to see more and more families become empowered in that they know that they can, they don't have to go to the store, the drug store for everything. That there's food medicines and plant medicines that they can find in their own yards or around the center. I think if families, you know, opening their minds to those habits, I think that will be really helpful. And then you know we're a very community based, so when things are done in groups, it's usually more successful. [twenty-eight-year-old Oneida woman with diabetic family members]

As Rosanna stated, the diabetes epidemic in Native Chicago cannot be treated as an independent health issue. To address improving diabetes care and prevention efforts in Chicago's Indigenous community, we must, as Rosanna explains, think more holistically about well-being. In this conclusion, I briefly outline the main findings of this book before describing what interview participants said they would like to see for the future. I situate these desires within scholarship that describes aims to decolonize health and increase collaborative efforts through participatory research to illustrate how these initiatives would benefit wellness program development in Chicago's Native community and meet the desires of the community.

Main Findings

While diabetes has been found in human populations for several millennia, cases of type 2 diabetes were rare in American Indian populations prior to the mid-twentieth century. Today Indigenous Americans have some of the highest rates of diabetes in the world. The majority of the research on this epidemic focuses on reservation populations. While rates of diabetes climbed in reservation areas, they also grew in cities, where most Native people live today. In this work, I have explored experiences with, understandings of, and care for diabetes in Chicago's Native community.

In doing so this work theorizes the relationship between human health and culture. I have demonstrated that history and society shape human health. The diabetes epidemic in Native North America is the embodiment of a long and continuing history of colonial oppression and forced migration. The epidemic status of diabetes in Native communities also shapes modern culture and society. I have described how Native identity is articulated through, and the intertribal community of Chicago is strengthened in, discourses of shared physiologies that represent a common evolutionary history. I have also shown how the shared work of diabetes care binds this intertribal community together, strengthening Indigenous Americans' ties in the city space.

Looking to the Future: A Call for Community-Engaged Efforts

The Indigenous peoples of the Americas, both urban and rural, face significant disparities in health in comparison to other racial and ethnic groups within the United States. Urban Native communities face these disparities while also being one of the most overlooked and underserved ethnic minority populations in the country. Urban Indigenous peoples and their health concerns are in need of and deserving of attention. By this I do not mean attention from paternalistic public-health do-gooders. Rather, what is needed is collaborative and community-engaged work that aims to decolonize health-care efforts by considering health and wellness more holistically.

According to Carolyn Smith-Morris, the biomedical system in which most Indigenous Americans receive their diabetes care is based on colonial structures, including those of capitalism, pharmaceutical markets, and racism.[1] To decolonize health care is to return to a more holistic view of wellness. In her autobiography, *The Scalpel and the Silver Bear*, Navajo surgeon Lori Arviso-Alvord describes her experiences of living and working across two worlds, those of her Navajo and her biomedical cultures. In the concluding chapter she outlines parameters for her idealized healing setting, a setting in which patients and healers are partners who listen to one another, where the whole of the person and their life is considered in both creating an understanding of what is ailing them and developing steps to take to improve wellness, and which equally considers and incorporates the voices of community members, traditional healers, and medical providers to meet these aims on a broader level.[2]

In recent decades participatory research has increasingly met with success in Indigenous communities and offers a realistic route to decolonizing health-care practices. Participatory research is a collaborative effort and reciprocal process whereby researchers and communities work together to develop research programs, collect data, and produce knowledge that is useful to both the researched community and intellectual audiences. Participatory research was developed in the 1970s with the goal of empowering communities through research.[3] I suggest that, for diabetes care, this focus on engaging the community to develop management as well as prevention programs is necessary, particularly because the vast majority of diabetes care and prevention work is done outside of clinical settings. Local community members know their own needs and capabilities best and engaging with local leaders will produce better long-term outcomes. Further, collaborative projects within Indigenous communities have demonstrated success in the past in both reservation and urban areas.[4]

While the focus of this research was documenting the experience of diabetes and its care, I concluded each of my interviews with the same question—what would you like to see happen for diabetes care and prevention in the future? Education was the top response. This ranged from education specifically about diabetes and healthy diets to more general education about living healthy lifestyles in a city space. Many focused on the importance of educating not only diabetics but the community at large. Educating the community more broadly was described as important because so much of the care work is done outside of homes and in communal spaces. Further, there was a great interest in the development of education programs that are directed to the whole family, with future generations in mind. Participants were thinking about teaching children to live a healthy lifestyle early in life to promote wellness, and perhaps prevent diabetes and other chronic diseases in the future.

Another common response to this question of what the community would like to see happen was the desire for more supported efforts from local organizations, particularly efforts that incorporate Indigenous traditions. These included hosting programs and events like diabetes talking circles, offering family cooking classes incorporating traditional foods, and organizing weight loss competitions. At the center of these responses was the desire for working together as a larger community and to have a bit of fun in the process.

Far more work is needed to meet the challenges faced by urban Indigenous communities in terms of health and well-being. I suggest that this work should (1) focus on collaboration and community empowerment, (2) consider wellness holistically, (3) aim to address issues of poverty, social inequality, and food insecurity, (4) incorporate Indigenous traditions in the urban space, and (5) find tangible ways to support Indigenous community centers, as they are vital to community wellness. Members of this community have highlighted the fact that the Indigenous peoples of the Americas are resilient. They will survive the diabetes epidemic, just as they have survived many other obstacles brought on by colonialism.

APPENDIX 1

Interview Participants

For this study, I completed 124 interviews with 97 participants. Interviewees identified themselves as citizens of American Indian Nations from across the United States and Canada, including the Apache, Akimel O'odham, Arikara, Assiniboine, Cherokee, Chippewa, Choctaw, Covelo, Dakota, Ho-Chunk, Lakota, Menominee, Meskwaki, Micmac, Navajo, Odawa, Ojibwe, Omaha, Oneida, Ponca, Potawatomi, Pueblo, Sac and Fox, Seneca, Sioux, and Stockbridge Nations.

The study comprised two types of interviews, namely, diabetes and oral history interviews. These included ninety-three interviews on diabetes and thirty-one oral history interviews with first and second generation relocatees to Chicago (see table 3). I conducted diabetes interviews between 2007 and 2013. These included forty-six interviews with forty people living with diabetes (fifteen men and twenty-five women), thirty interviews with thirty family members of diabetics (thirteen men and seventeen women), and seventeen interviews with thirteen medical professionals (one man and twelve women, five self-identified as Native and eight as non-Native). Additionally, between 2012 and 2017 I conducted thirty-one oral history interviews to learn more about Chicago's Native community and its history. Interviewees included nine men and twenty women who were between the ages of fifty and eighty-seven and who had moved (or their parents had moved) to a city during the era of the federal relocation program.

Table 3. Interview participants

	Diabetes interviews	Caregiver interviews	Biomedical provider interviews	Oral history interviews
GENDER				
Male	15	13	1	9
Female	25	17	12	20
AGE				
18–30	4	7	3	0
31–45	8	9	2	0
46–60	13	13	5	12
61–75	13	1	3	12
76+	2	0	0	5
HAS DIABETES				
Yes	40	0	3	14
No	0	30	10	15
YEARS WITH DIABETES				
Less than 1 year	8	-	-	-
1–2	5	-	-	-
3–5	10	-	-	-
6–10	4	-	-	-
11–15	5	-	-	-
16–20	1	-	-	-
21 or more	7	-	-	-
TYPE OF CARE PROVIDER				
Physician	-	-	1	-
Dietician	-	-	1	-
Nurse	-	-	7	-
Community health worker	-	-	4	-

WORKS PRIMARILY WITH NATIVE POPULATION				
Yes	-	-	10	-
No	-	-	3	-

YEAR MOVED TO CHICAGO				
1951–60	-	-	-	8
1961–70	-	-	-	5
1971–80	-	-	-	5
1981–90	-	-	-	2
Born in Chicago	-	-	-	9

APPENDIX 2

Sample Questions

Diabetes Interview Sample Questions
How would you define diabetes?
Why do people develop diabetes?
How does diabetes affect someone's life?
How can diabetes be treated?
What challenges are there, if any, to diabetes care?
What would you like to see happen for diabetes care and
prevention in the future?

Ethnohistory Interview Questions
How long have you lived in Chicago?
What brought you to the city?
Where else have you lived?
What has life been like in Chicago?
Have you been involved in Chicago's Native community?

APPENDIX 3

Research Approval

This study was approved by the Social and Behavioral Sciences Internal Review Board (IRB) of the University of Wisconsin Madison under protocol number SE-2009-0188, the Minimal Risk Internal Review Board of the University of Wisconsin Madison under protocol number 2012-0345, and the Institutional Review Board of Northwestern University under protocol number 00201965. In accordance with the requirements of the IRB, throughout this work I refer to participants using pseudonyms. These pseudonyms were randomly chosen using the website fakenamegenerator.com. All tribal affiliations are those named by the participants, using the spelling they provided. Ages associated with participants are their age at the time of the interview.

NOTES

Introduction

1. All names of research participants are pseudonyms. The age listed is the age the person was at the time of the interview. Throughout, the tribes noted are the Indigenous American nations the interviewee noted being descended from.

2. Jones, "Death, Uncertainty, and Rhetoric," 25–37; Thornton, *American Indian Holocaust*, 44–47.

3. Centers for Disease Control and Prevention, "National Diabetes Statistics," 4.

4. West, "Diabetes in American Indian," 841–42.

5. Centers for Disease Control and Prevention, "National Diabetes Statistics," 4; West, "Diabetes in American Indian," 841–47; Knowler et al., "Diabetes Mellitus in the Pima Indians: Incidence, Risk Factors and Pathogenesis," 2.

6. Norris, Vines, and Hoeffel, "American Indian and Alaska Native Population," 12.

7. Kramer, "Health and Aging," 284; Rhoades, Roubideaux, and Buchwald, "Diabetes Care," 574.

8. American Indian Center of Chicago, "Mission Statement."

9. Deloria, *Custer Died for Your Sins*; King, "Here Come the Anthros"; Mihesuah, *So You Want to Write*; Smith, *Decolonizing Methodologies*.

10. I occasionally offered to drive senior community members home from center events. Furthermore, from 2012 through 2014 I occasionally commuted to Chicago from my home in Northwest Indiana with a community member who lived nearby.

11. de Cora, "Diabetic Plague," 11–13; Cantrell, "Access and Barriers," 65–67; Jackson, "Diet, Culture, and Diabetes," 381–406; Mihesuah, "Decolonizing Our Diets," 819–24.

12. Evaneshko, "Presenting Complaints," 357–77; Garcia-Smith, "Gila River Diabetes Prevention," 471–94; Hickey and Carter, "Cultural Barriers," 453–70; Roy, "Diabetes and Identity," 167–86.

13. Garro, "Intracultural Variation," 399–406; Garro, "Remembering What One Knows," 296–308; Garro and Lang, "Explanations of Diabetes," 293–328; Lang, "Talking about a New Illness," 203–30; Smith-Morris, "Diagnostic Controversy," 160–66; Weiner, "Ethnogenetics," 160–71; Weiner, "Interpreting Ideas," 108–33.

14. Bruna, "Religious Gardens," 126–36; Olson, "Applying Medical Anthropology," 188–95; Olson, "Meeting the Challenges," 163–84; Smith-Morris, " Community Participation," 96–103; Wilson et al., "Community Approaches," 495–503.

15. Forbes, "The Urban Tradition," 15–41; Snipp, "Sociological Perspectives," 358; Sorkin, *Urban American Indian*, 26–27.

16. Arndt, "Contrary to Our Way"; Jackson, *Our Elders Lived It*; Lobo, "Is Urban a Person"; Ramirez, *Native Hubs*.

17. de Cora, "Diabetic Plague," 11–13; Cantrell, "Access and Barriers," 65–67; Jackson, "Diet, Culture, and Diabetes," 381–406.

18. Garro, "Remembering What One Knows," 296–308; Hunt, "Moral Reasoning," 302–9; Sahota, "Genetic Histories," 828–35.

1. Chicago's Indigenous Population

1. Lazewski, "American Indian Migration," 25 and 51; Ramirez, *Native Hubs*, 55–56.

2. American Indian Center of Chicago, "Mission Statement"; United States Census Bureau, "ACS Demographic."

3. Low, *Imprints*, xi; Vogel, "Indian Place Names," 63–65.

4. Vogel, "Indian Place Names," 63–65.

5. Beck, *Chicago American Indian*; Low, *Imprints*, 22–32.

6. Low, *Imprints*.

7. Cattelino, *High Stakes*, 175; Levinson, "Explanation for the Oneida-Colonist Alliance," 265–89; Ricciardelli, "Adoption of White Agriculture," 312–13; Ritzenthaler, "Oneida Indians," 1–5; Thornton, *American Indian Holocaust*, 47–49.

8. Thornton, *American Indian Holocaust*, 44–47.

9. Crosby, "Virgin Soil Epidemics"; Jones, "Death, Uncertainty, and Rhetoric."

10. Jones, "Death, Uncertainty, and Rhetoric," 16–37.

11. Jones, "Death, Uncertainty, and Rhetoric," 25–37; Pearson, "Lewis Cass," 12–23; Thornton, *American Indian Holocaust*, 44–53.

12. Pearson, "Lewis Cass," 12–23.

13. Goldberg-Ambrose, "Native Americans and Tribal Members," 1130–31; Iverson, *We Are Still Here*, 5–7; Maybury-Lewis, *Indigenous Peoples*, 48; Straus and Valentino, "Retribalization," par. 6.

14. Southall, "Illusion of Tribe," 28–36.

15. Grinnell, *Cheyenne Indians*, 2–3.

16. Goldberg-Ambrose, "Native Americans and Tribal Members," 1123–48.

17. U.S. Const. art. 1, § 8, cl. 3.

18. U.S. Const., art. 6, cl. 2.

19. Deloria and Lytle, *Nations Within*, 16–17.

20. McCarthy, "Bureau of Indian Affairs," 19–25.

21. Cave, "Abuse of Power," 1330–53; Trafzer, *As Long as the Grass*, 148–49; Wilkinson and Briggs, "Evolution of Termination Policy," 141.

22. Cave, "Abuse of Power," 1330–53; Iverson and Roessel, *Diné*, 51–65; Low, *Imprints*, 30; Sturm, *Blood Politics*, 11–14 and 62–68.

23. Neils, *Reservation to City*, 5.

24. Clark, *Lone Wolf v. Hitchcock*, 38–43; Biolsi, "Birth of the Reservation," 30–35; Wilkinson and Briggs, "Evolution of Termination Policy," 142–43.

25. Lajimodiere, "Healing Journey," 5–19; Lomawaima, "Domesticity in the Federal Indian Schools," 227–31; Chicago American Indian Oral History Pilot Project 1983–1985, box 2, folders 1 and 6, and box 3, folder 9.

26. Cattelino, *High Stakes*, 161–92; Goldberg-Ambrose, "Native Americans and Tribal Members," 1123–48. Jarding, "Tribal-State Relations," 298–302; Rand and Light, "Do 'Fish and Chips' Mix," 129–42.

27. Meriam and Work, *Problem of Indian Administration*; Trafzer, *As Long as the Grass*, 345–56.

28. Forbes, "The Urban Tradition," 15–41; Low, *Imprints*, xi; Thrush, *Native Seattle*, 3–16.

29. Meriam and Work, *Problem of Indian Administration*, 667; LaPier and Beck, "One-Man Relocation," 19.

30. Rosenthal, *Reimagining Indian Country*, 11–22; Intertribal Friendship House and Lobo, *Urban Voices*, 1–16; LaPier and Beck, "One-Man Relocation," 18.

31. LaPier and Beck, "One-Man Relocation," 20.

32. Meriam and Work, *Problem of Indian Administration*, 669–70.

33. LaPier and Beck, "One-Man Relocation," 23–24 and 28–31.

34. LaPier and Beck, "One-Man Relocation," 33.

35. Arndt, "Relocation's Imagined Landscape," 159–72; Jackson, *Our Elders Lived It*, 48–49; Miller, "Willing Workers," 51–76.

36. Jackson, *Our Elders Lived It*, 48–49.

37. Miller, *Indians on the Move*, 42–67.

38. Lazewski, "American Indian Migration," 33.

39. Fixico, *Termination and Relocation*, 21; Iverson, *We Are Still Here*, 119–35.

40. Neils, *Reservation to City*, 6–7.

41. Jaeger et al., *Tribal Nations*; Lewis, "Still Native," 217.

42. Fixico, *Termination and Relocation*, 21–44; Iverson, *We Are Still Here*, 126; Neils, *Reservation to City*, 6.

43. Cowger, *National Congress*, 100; Fixico, *Termination and Relocation*, 33–34; Iverson, *We Are Still Here*, 122.

44. Iverson, *We Are Still Here*, 122.

45. Fixico, *Termination and Relocation*, 21–44 and 183–86.

46. Philp, "Stride toward Freedom," 178.

47. Bennett et al., "Relocation," 164–66; Burt, *Tribalism in Crisis*, 7.

48. Fixico, *Termination and Relocation*, 94–99.

49. House Concurrent Resolution 108, *U.S. Statutes at Large* 67 (1953), B132.

50. Cowger, *National Congress*, 99–125; Fixico, *Termination and Relocation*, 180–81.

51. Burt, *Tribalism in Crisis*, 25.

52. The mandatory states and territories included California, Minnesota, Oregon, Nebraska, Wisconsin, and the Alaskan territory. Burt, *Tribalism in Crisis*, 25.

53. Burt, *Tribalism in Crisis*, 108; Philp, "Stride toward Freedom," 179–80.

54. Jackson, *Our Elders Lived It*, 27; Miller, "Willing Workers," 51–76; Rosenthal, *Reimagining Indian Country*, 11–30.

55. Chicago American Indian Oral History Pilot Project, "Native Voices," 60–70; Garcia, "Urbanization of Rural Population," 194–95; Philp, "Stride toward Freedom," 175–77.

56. Lazewski, "American Indian Migration," 32.

57. Neils, *Reservation to City*, 46–47; Sorkin, *Urban American Indian*, 25.

58. Watkins and Sherk, "Who Serves," 10.

59. Chicago American Indian Oral History Pilot Project, "Native Voices," 29–40.

60. Arends, "Socio-Cultural Study," ch. 2; Fixico, *Termination and Relocation*, 136; Intertribal Friendship House and Lobo, *Urban Voices*, 19.

61. Burt, *Tribalism in Crisis*, 6–7; Fixico, *Termination and Relocation*, 134–35; Iverson and Roessel, *Diné*, 193–94; King, "Urbanization"; Rosenthal, *Reimagining Indian Country*, 52.

62. Fixico, *Termination and Relocation*, 136; Intertribal Friendship House and Lobo, *Urban Voices*, 19.

63. Neils, *Reservation to City*, 58–63; Rosenthal, *Reimagining Indian Country*, 11–30.

64. Neils, *Reservation to City*, 91.

65. Jackson, "Place Where I Can," 36.

66. United States Bureau of Indian Affairs, "Indian Relocation Records."

67. United States Bureau of Indian Affairs, "Brief History," 2.

68. United States Bureau of Indian Affairs, "Brief History," 1.

69. United States Bureau of Indian Affairs, "Brief History," 1.

70. Chicago American Indian Oral History Pilot Project, "Native Voices," 18–19.

71. Iverson, *We Are Still Here*, 134; Iverson, "Knowing the Land," 69.

72. "Report Indian Families Like Suburban Life: Making Good on Jobs in City Area," *Chicago Daily Tribune*, June 17, 1957, 23.

73. Iverson, "Knowing the Land," 67–70; Burt, *Tribalism in Crisis*, 57; Chicago American Indian Oral History Pilot Project, "Native Voices."

74. Arends, "Socio-Cultural Study," ch. 2.

75. Saint Augustine's, "Records," box 5; Rosenthal, *Reimagining Indian Country*, 56.

76. Snipp, "Sociological Perspectives," 358; Sorkin, *Urban American Indian*, 26–27.

77. Sorkin, *Urban American Indian*, 25.

78. Norris et al., "American Indian and Alaska Native Population," 12.

79. Chicago American Indian Oral History Pilot Project, "Project Records," boxes 2–3.

80. Sorkin, *Urban American Indian*, 25.

81. Sorkin, *Urban American Indian*, 27.

82. Arends, "Socio-Cultural Study," ch. 4; Arndt, "Relocation's Imagined Landscape," 159–72; United States Bureau of Indian Affairs, "Indian Relocation Records."

83. Arends, "Socio-Cultural Study," ch. 4.

84. Sorkin, *American Indians and Federal Aid*, 8.

85. de Cora, "Diabetic Plague," 11–13; Cantrell, "Access and Barriers," 65–67; Jackson, "Diet, Culture, and Diabetes," 381–406; Mihesuah, "Decolonizing Our Diets," 819–24.

86. Chicago American Indian Oral History Pilot Project, "Project Records," boxes 2–3.

87. I asked interviewees about the most pressing health and social concerns of Chicago's Native population. Diabetes, alcoholism, poor dental health, and unemployment were the four most frequently named issues.

88. Lazewski, "American Indian Migration," 47–48; Rosenthal, *Reimagining Indian Country*, 86; Snipp, "Sociological Perspectives," 360–61.

89. LaGrand, *Indian Metropolis*, 233–44; Wilson, "Chicago Indian Village," 212–19.

90. Correspondence from Gerard Littman to Father Peter Powell, Saint Augustine's, "Records," box 5.

91. Blackhawk, "Carry On from Here," 16–30; Snyder, "Kinship, Friendship, and Enclave," 117–29; Intertribal Friendship House and Lobo, *Urban Voices*; Chicago American Indian Oral History Pilot Project, "Native Voices"; Arndt, "Relocation's Imagined Landscape," 159–72; Bennett et al., "Relocation," 161–73.

92. Blackhawk, "Carry On from Here," 22; Intertribal Friendship House and Lobo, *Urban Voices*, 24; Rosenthal, *Reimagining Indian Country*, 56–57.

93. Sorkin, *Urban American Indian*, 72–74.

94. Eagle, "Urban Indians and the Occupation," 52–73; Willard, "Indian Newspapers," 91–97.

95. Chicago American Indian Oral History Pilot Project, "Native Voices"; Lazewski, "American Indian Migration," 41–45; Neils, *Reservation to City*, 94; Sorkin, *Urban American Indian*, 72–74.

96. LaGrand, "Indian Work and Indian Neighborhoods," 207.

97. Chicago American Indian Oral History Pilot Project, "Native Voices."

98. Arends, "Socio-Cultural Study," ch. 2; Bennett et al., "Relocation," 161–73; Fixico, *Termination and Relocation*, 140–50; Sorkin, *American Indians and Federal Aid*, 8.

99. Garcia, "Urbanization of Rural Population," 201–4; LaGrand, *Indian Metropolis*, 233–44; Wilson, "Chicago Indian Village," 212–19.

100. Garcia, "Urbanization of Rural Population," 196–97.

101. Burt, *Tribalism in Crisis*, 57.

2. Native Chicago

1. Straus and Valentino, "Retribalization," par. 23.

2. Meyer, "American Indian Blood Quantum," 234.

3. Garroutte, "Racial Formation of American Indians," 224–26; Harmon, "Tribal Enrollment Councils," 177–90; Meyer, "American Indian Blood Quantum Requirements";

Tallbear, "DNA, Blood, and Racializing the Tribe," 88–93; Tallbear, *Native American DNA*, 45–66.

4. Garroutte, "Racial Formation of American Indians," 224–26; Tallbear, "DNA, Blood, and Racializing the Tribe," 82–83.

5. Harmon, "Tribal Enrollment Councils," 180–81; Straus and Valentino, "Retribalization," par. 6.

6. Tallbear, "DNA, Blood, and Racializing the Tribe," 89.

7. Harmon, "Tribal Enrollment Councils," 175–200.

8. Tallbear, *Native American DNA*, 120–21.

9. Weaver, "Indigenous Identity," 244–47.

10. Clifford, *Predicament of Culture*, 277–346.

11. Hill and Wilson, "Identity Politics," 2.

12. Oritz, "Indian or Not," 437–42.

13. Sturm, *Blood Politics*, 18–20 and 161–65.

14. Quoted in Zhao, "Self-Identification."

15. Cattelino, *High Stakes*, 59–94; Garbarino, "Life in the City," 168–205; Goldberg-Ambrose, "Native Americans and Tribal Members," 1130–31; Gonzales, "(Re)Articulation of American Indian Identity," 199–225; Lobo, "Is Urban a Person," 89–102; Sturm, *Blood Politics*, 29–44.

16. Connerton, *How Societies Remember*, 1–40; Hill and Wilson, "Identity Politics," 2.

17. Guss, "Selling of San Juan," 451–73; Guss, "Cimarrones, Theater and the State," 180–92.

18. Simon, "Contesting Formosa," 109–31.

19. Webster, "All the Former Cats and Stomps," 63–67.

20. Jackson, *Our Elders Lived It*, 166.

21. Lobo, "Is Urban a Person," 89–102.

22. LaGrand, "Indian Work and Indian Neighborhoods," 202–7.

23. Gonzales, "(Re)Articulation of American Indian Identity," 199–225; Nagel, "American Indian Ethnic Renewal," 947–65.

24. Snipp, "Sociological Perspectives," 357–60.

25. Jackson, "Hole in Our Heart," 227–54.

26. Paredes, "Toward a Reconceptualization," 256–71.

27. Ramirez, *Natives Hubs*, 58–199.

28. Viruell-Fuentes, "My Heart Is Always There," 335–62.

29. Bourdieu, "Taste of Luxury," 72–78; Caplan, "Approaches to the Study of Food," 1–31; Roy, "Diabetes and Identity," 167–86; Sutton, *Remembrance of Repasts*.

30. Caplan, "Approaches to the Study of Food," 1–31; Sutton, *Remembrance of Repasts*.

31. Frybread is considered by community members as a Native food, but not a traditional Native food, as it was developed in the colonial era.

32. Arndt, "Nation in the City," 337–41; Straus and Valentino, "Retribalization," par. 17.

33. Arndt, "Nation in the City," 337–41.

34. Spicer, "Indian Identity," 47.

35. Cattelino, *High Stakes*, 69–73.

36. Low, *Imprints*, 147.

37. Suzukovich, "Seen and Unseen."

38. Kiesling, "Now I Gotta Watch," 250–53; West and Zimmerman, "Doing Gender."

39. Herzfeld, *Body Impolitic*, 60.

40. Lobo, "Is Urban a Person," 89–102.

41. Clifford, *Predicament of Culture*, 277–346.

42. Abdelhady, "Beyond Home/Host Networks."

43. Deloria, *Indians in Unexpected Places*, 3–11.

44. Beck, "Chicago American Indian Community," 45–47; Deloria, *Indians in Unexpected Places*, 3–11; Intertribal Friendship House and Lobo, *Urban Voices*; Weibel-Orlando, *Indian Country, L.A.*

45. St. Augustine's Center for the American Indian closed permanently in the late 2010s, after having served the community for more than sixty years.

46. Chicago American Indian Oral History Pilot Project, "Project Records," box 2, folder 8.

47. Ono, "I am a Denver Indian," 83–91; Snipp, "Sociological Perspectives," 359–60.

48. Krouse, "Traditional Iroquois Socials," 400–408; Suzukovich, "Seen and Unseen."

49. Ramirez, *Native Hubs*, 98–100 and 134.

50. American Indian Center of Chicago, "Statement on Blackhawks."

3. Diabetes among Indigenous Americans

1. Aretæus, Adams, and Sydenham Society, 338–40; von Klein, "Medical Features of the Papyrus Ebers," 1930; Galen, *Galen on Diseases*, 200; Papaspyros, *History of Diabetes*; Sanders, "Thebes to Toronto"; Schneider, "Diabetes through the Ages," 1394–95.

2. Joslin, "Universality of Diabetes," 2035–37; West, "Diabetes in American Indian," 841–42.

3. Knowler et al., "Diabetes Mellitus in the Pima: Incidence, Risk Factors and Pathogenesis," 2; Pavkov et al., "Changing Patterns of Type 2 Diabetes," 1758–63; Szathmáry, "Non-Insulin Dependent Diabetes," 459–61; West, "Diabetes in American Indian," 841–47.

4. Centers for Disease Control and Prevention, "National Diabetes Statistics," 4; Centers for Disease Control and Prevention, "2017 Diabetes Report," 3.

5. Centers for Disease Control and Prevention, "2017 Diabetes Report," 7–8; Spanakis and Golden, "Race/Ethnic Difference in Diabetes," 3–6.

6. Papaspyros, *History of Diabetes*, 1–15; Sanders, "Thebes to Toronto"; Schneider, "Diabetes through the Ages," 1394–95; Feudtner, "Diabetes," 397.

7. Sigma Type Diabetes Consortium, "Sequence Variants."

8. Papaspyros, *History of Diabetes*, 4; von Klein, "Medical Features of The Papyrus Ebers," 1930; Christopoulou-Aletra and Paparamidou, "'Diabetes' as Described," 892.

9. Gemmill, "Greek Concept of Diabetes," 1034; Papaspyros, *History of Diabetes*, 5–11; Schneider, "Diabetes through the Ages," 1394–95; Morgan, *Diabetes Mellitus*, 4.

10. Christopoulou-Aletra and Paparamidou, "'Diabetes' as Described," 893; Schneider, "Diabetes through the Ages," 1394; Gemmill, "Greek Concept of Diabetes," 1035.

11. Gemmill, "Greek Concept of Diabetes," 1033; Papaspyros, *History of Diabetes*; Sanders, "Thebes to Toronto," 57; Schneider, "Diabetes through the Ages," 1394; Henschen, "On the Term Diabetes," 190.

12. Aretæus, "On Diabetes," 6.

13. Aretæus, "On Diabetes," 3.

14. Aretæus, "On Diabetes," 3.

15. Gemmill, "Greek Concept of Diabetes," 1035.

16. Henschen, "On the Term Diabetes," 192.

17. Henschen, "On the Term Diabetes," 192; Sanders, "Thebes to Toronto," 57; Schneider, "Diabetes through the Ages," 1394.

18. Henschen, "On the Term Diabetes," 191–92; Papaspyros, *History of Diabetes*, 5.

19. Clarke and Foster, "History of Blood Glucose Meters," 83–84.

20. Papaspyros, *History of Diabetes*.

21. Feudtner, "Diabetes," 397; Papaspyros, *History of Diabetes*.

22. Knorr Cetina, *Epistemic Cultures*; Latour and Woolgar, *Laboratory Life*; Pickering, *Mangle of Practice*.

23. Clarke et al., "Biomedicalization," 162–63.

24. See for example Fullwiley, *Enculturated Gene*; Livingston, *Improvising Medicine*; Lock and Nguyen, *Anthropology of Biomedicine*; Wendland, *Heart for the Work*.

25. Epstein, *Inclusion*, 1–16 and 30–52; Foucault, *Discipline and Punish*; Lock and Nguyen, *Anthropology of Biomedicine*, 32–56; Rose, *Politics of Life Itself*, 3–4.

26. Clarke et al., "Biomedicalization," 173–76; Lock and Nguyen, *Anthropology of Biomedicine*, 15–31; Rose, "Human Sciences in a Biological Age," 3–34.

27. Lock and Nguyen, *Anthropology of Biomedicine*, 56.

28. Papaspyros, *History of Diabetes*; Rosenfeld, "Insulin," 2271–72.

29. See Rosenfeld, "Insulin," for a description of the scientific history, partnership, and later rivalry of Fredrick Banting and John James Rickard Macleod in this process.

30. Papaspyros, *History of Diabetes*; Rosenfeld, "Insulin," 2283–84.

31. Rosenfeld, "Insulin," 2280.

32. American Diabetes Association, "Executive Summary," 581.

33. Martin, "Woman in the Flexible Body," 97–115; Scheper-Hughes and Lock, "Mindful Body," 22–23.

34. Rapp, "Real-Time Fetus," 31–48.

35. Lock, *Twice Dead*, 32–129; Mol, *Body Multiple*, 29–52.

36. Mol, *Body Multiple*.

37. Mol, "What Diagnostic Devices Do," 9–22.

38. Clarke and Foster, "History of Blood Glucose Meters," 83–93.

39. American Diabetes Association, "Executive Summary"; Himsworth, "Diabetes Mellitus"; Neel, "Thrifty Genotype Revisited."

40. Centers for Disease Control and Prevention, "2017 Diabetes Report," 7–8; Fagot-Campagna, Narayan, and Imperatore, "Type 2 Diabetes in Children," 377–78; Spanakis and Golden, "Race/Ethnic Difference in Diabetes," 3–6.

41. For examples see American Diabetes Association, "Executive Summary."

42. Documented in Hrdlička, *Physiological and Medical Observations*, 182.

43. Joslin, "Universality of Diabetes," 2035–37.

44. West, "Diabetes in American Indian," 841–42.

45. West, "Diabetes in American Indian," 841–47; Wiedman, "Native American Embodiment," 598–603.

46. Indian Health Service, "Gold Book."

47. Centers for Disease Control and Prevention, "National Diabetes Statistics," 4; Gallo and Schell, "Height, Weight, and Body Mass Index," 269–79; Gilliland et al., "Temporal Trends," 422–31; Gohdes, "Diabetes in American Indians," 609–13; Knowler et al., "Diabetes Mellitus in the Pima: Incidence, Risk Factors and Pathogenesis," 2; Kramer, "Health and Aging," 284; Pavkov et al., "Changing Patterns of Type 2 Diabetes," 1758–63; Pettitt et al., "Mortality as a Function," 359–66; Rhoades, Roubideaux, and Buchwald, "Diabetes Care," 574; Rith-Najarian, Valway, and Ghodes, "Diabetes in a Northern Minnesota Chippewa Tribe," 266–70; Young, "Diabetes among Canadian Indians and Inuit," 21–40.

48. Parry, "Pacific Islanders Pay Heavy Price," 484–85.

49. Kramer, "Health and Aging," 284; Rhoades, Roubideaux, and Buchwald, "Diabetes Care," 574.

50. Centers for Disease Control and Prevention, "National Diabetes Statistics," 4.

51. Foucault, *Discipline and Punish*.

52. Grinker, *Unstrange Minds*, 2–6.

53. Whitmarsh, *Biomedical Ambiguity*, 69–97.

54. Ferzacca, *Healing the Modern*, 52–54.

55. Neel, "Diabetes Mellitus: A 'Thrifty' Genotype," 353–62; Neel, "Thrifty Genotype Revisited," 283–93; Neel, "'Thrifty Genotype' in 1998," 2–9.

56. Knowler et al., "Diabetes mellitus in the Pima Indians: Genetic and Evolutionary Considerations," 113. Knowler et al., "Diabetes Mellitus in the Pima Indians: Incidence, Risk Factors and Pathogenesis," 20; Pettitt et al., "Mortality as a Function," 364–65.

57. Neel, "'Thrifty Genotype' in 1998," 2–9.

58. Allen and Cheer, "The Non-Thrifty Genotype," 831–42.

59. Ozanne and Hales, "Thrifty Yes, Genetic No," 485–87; Southam et al., "Is the Thrifty Genotype Hypothesis Supported," 1846–51.

60. Ali, "Genetics of Type 2 Diabetes," 115–18; Udler, "Type 2 Diabetes," 3–6.

61. Hales and Barker, "Type 2 (Non-Insulin-Dependent) Diabetes Mellitus," 597.

62. Benyshek, "The 'Early Life' Origins," 80–89; Casazza et al., "Beyond Thriftiness," 182; Vaag et al., "Thrifty Phenotype Hypothesis Revisited," 2085–88.

63. Allen and Cheer, "The Non-Thrifty Genotype," 831–42; Birnbaum, "Rejoinder," 129–34; Gilliland et al., "Temporal Trends," 422–31; Justice, "History of Diabetes,"

69–128; Pettitt et al., "Mortality as a Function," 359–66; Szathmáry, "Non-Insulin Dependent Diabetes," 459–76; Szathmáry and Ferrell, "Glucose Level, Acculturation," 333–36; Wiedman, "Globalizing the Chronicities"; Wiedman, "Native American Embodiment," 595–606; Young, "Diabetes among Canadian Indians and Inuit," 21–40.

64. Buchanan, "(How) Can We Prevent," 1502–7; Fretts et al., "Physical Activity and Incident Diabetes," 632–39; Gallo and Schell, "Height, Weight, and Body Mass Index," 269–79; Hamilton, Hamilton, and Zderic, "Role of Low Energy Expenditure," 2655–67; Knowler et al., "Diabetes Incidence in Pima Indians: Contributions of Obesity," 144–56; Kriska et al., "Physical Activity, Obesity, and the Incidence of Type 2 Diabetes," 669–75; Pettitt et al., "Mortality as a Function," 359–66.

65. Schulz, "Traditional Environment Protects," 68–70.

66. Whyte, "The Publics of the New Public Health," 187–207.

67. Ferreira and Lang, "Introduction," 3–32; Scheper-Hughes, "Forward," xvii–xxi.

68. de Cora, "Diabetic Plague," 11–13.

69. Jackson, "Diet, Culture, and Diabetes," 388.

70. de Cora, "Diabetic Plague," 11–13.

71. Cantrell, "Access and Barriers," 65–67.

72. Justice, "History of Diabetes," 69–128.

73. Galtung, "Violence, Peace, and Peace Research," 170.

74. For the full range of discussions of structural violence in Paul Farmer's work, see *Infections and Inequalities*, *Pathologies of Power*, and "On Suffering and Structural Violence."

4. Diabetes in Native Chicago

1. These dark patches of skin on the neck and/or underarm are known as acanthosis nigricans in the biomedical community—described in that context as an early sign of insulin resistance, documented in Hearst et al., "Co-Occurrence of Obesity," 346–52.

2. Chicago American Indian Oral History Pilot Project, "Project Records," box 3, folder 12, page 15.

3. Schutz, *Collected Papers I*, 71–76.

4. Schutz, *On Phenomenology*, 72–77.

5. George, *Picturing Islam*, 4.

6. Jackson, *Minima Ethnographica*, 3–35; Schutz, *Collected Papers I*, 208–20; Schutz, *On Phenomenology*, 72–73; Williams, *Marxism and Literature*, 128–32.

7. Dumit, *Drugs for Life*; Klawiter, "Regulatory Shifts," 432–60; Petersen and Lupton, *New Public Health*.

8. Rose, *Politics of Life Itself*, 10.

9. Sahota, "Genetic Histories," 829.

10. Niehoff, "Discussion," 244–53.

11. Crapanzano, *Tuhami*.

12. Benedict, "Anthropology and the Abnormal."

13. Broom and Whittaker, "Controlling Diabetes," 2371–82; Whyte, "The Publics of the New Public Health," 187–207.

14. Bordo, *Unbearable Weight*; Counihan, *Anthropology of Food and Body*.

15. Broom and Whittaker, "Controlling Diabetes," 2371–82; Ferzacca, "'Actually, I Don't Feel That Bad,'" 28–50.

16. Conklin, "Hanunóo Color Categories," 339–34.

17. Rosaldo, "Metaphors and Folk Classification," 83–99.

18. Tsing, *Friction*, 193.

19. Bowker and Star, *Sorting Things Out*, 5.

20. Firth, "Twins, Birds and Vegetables," 1–17.

21. Hacking, "Making Up People," 150–63.

22. Frake, "Diagnosis of Disease," 113–32.

23. Hunt and Arar, "Analytical Framework for Contrasting," 347–67.

24. Bowker and Star, *Sorting Things Out*, 53–106.

25. Kreiner and Hunt, "Pursuit of Preventive Care," 876.

26. Dumit, *Drugs for Life*.

5. Local Understandings

1. Hunt, "Moral Reasoning," 302–9.

2. Sahota, "Genetic Histories," 828–35.

3. Hunt, "Moral Reasoning," 302–9; Sahota, "Genetic Histories," 828–35.

4. Garro, "Remembering What One Knows," 296–308.

5. McCombie, "Folk Flu," 27–43.

6. Mol, *Body Multiple*, 29–52.

7. Weiner, "Ethnogenetics," 160–71; Weiner, "Interpreting Ideas," 108–33.

8. Sahota, "Genetic Histories," 828–35.

9. Garro and Lang, "Explanations of Diabetes," 293–328.

10. Mihesuah, *Recovering Our Ancestors' Gardens*.

11. Centers for Disease Control and Prevention, "National Diabetes Statistics," 4; de Cora, "Diabetic Plague," 11–13; Indian Health Service, "Gold Book"; Wiedman, "Globalizing the Chronicities."

12. Fine, "Towards a Political Economy of Food," 538–39.

13. Cantrell, "Access and Barriers," 65–67; de Cora, "Diabetic Plague," 11–13; Jackson, "Diet, Culture, and Diabetes," 388; Justice, "History of Diabetes," 69–128.

14. Lang, "'In Their Tellings,'" 52–71; Lang, "Talking about a New Illness," 203–30.

15. Rock, "Sweet Blood and Social Suffering," 131–74.

16. Scheder, "Sickly-Sweet Harvest," 251–77.

17. Poss and Jezewski, "Role and Meaning of *Susto*," 360–77.

18. Thompson and Gifford, "Trying to Keep a Balance," 1457–72.

19. Ferzacca, *Healing the Modern*, 4.

20. Mendenhall et al., "Speaking through Diabetes," 220–39.

21. Schoenberg et al., "Situating Stress," 94–113.

22. Willis and Pordage, *Dr. Willis's Practice*, 72–76.

23. Björntorp, "Abdominal Obesity"; Björntorp, "Visceral Fat Accumulation"; Björntorp, "Body Fat Distribution"; Björntorp, "Do Stress Reactions Cause."

24. Pickup and Crook, "Is Type II Diabetes Mellitus."

25. Hartman and Gone, "American Indian Historical Trauma," 274–75.

26. Skinner, Manikkam, and Guerrero-Bosagna, "Epigenetic Transgenerational Actions," 214–22.

27. Matthews and Phillips, "Minireview," 7–13.

6. Care in the Context of Chronicity

1. American Indian Health Service of Chicago has since moved further west in the city to be nearer larger numbers of the population.

2. Becker, *Disrupted Lives*, 4–17.

3. Broom and Whittaker, "Controlling Diabetes," 2371–82.

4. For examples, see Pearson, "Lewis Cass"; Amy Harmon, "Tribe Wins Fight to Limit Research of its DNA," *New York Times*, April 21, 2010, https://www.nytimes.com/2010/04/22/us/22dna.html; Volscho, "Sterilization Racism," 17–31.

5. Heinemann, "For the Sake of Others," 66–84.

6. Seligman et al., "Self-Care and Subjectivity," 68–70.

7. Hunleth, "Children's Roles in Tuberculosis."

8. Livingston, *Improvising Medicine*, 6.

9. Olesen, "Caregiving, Ethical and Informal."

10. Mol, *Logic of Care*.

11. Fullwiley, *Enculturated Gene*, 46–57.

12. Guell, "Self-Care at the Margins."

Conclusion

1. Smith-Morris, "Bhabha in the Clinic," 49.

2. Alvord and Van Pelt, *The Scalpel and the Silver Bear*, 184–96.

3. Park, "What Is Participatory Research."

4. Macaulay et al., "Participatory Research"; Parker, "CBPR Principles"; Potvin et al., "Implementing Participatory Intervention"; Whitewater et al., "Flexible Roles."

BIBLIOGRAPHY

Abdelhady, Dalia. "Beyond Home/Host Networks: Forms of Solidarity among Lebanese Immigrants in a Global Era." *Identities: Global Studies in Culture and Power* 13, no. 3 (2006): 427–53. https://doi.org/10.1080/10702890600839595.

Ali, Omar. "Genetics of Type 2 Diabetes." *World Journal of Diabetes* 4, no. 4 (August 2013): 114–23. https://doi.org/10.4239/wjd.v4.i4.114.

Allen, John S., and Susan M. Cheer. "The Non-Thrifty Genotype." *Current Anthropology* 37, no. 5 (December 1996): 831–42. https://doi.org/10.1086/204566.

Alvord, Lori Arviso, and Elizabeth Cohen Van Pelt. *The Scalpel and the Silver Bear: The First Navajo Woman Surgeon Combines Western Medicine and Traditional Healing.* Des Plaines IL: Bantam Books, 1999.

American Diabetes Association. "Executive Summary: Standards of Medical Care in Diabetes—2014." *Diabetes Care* 37, supplement 1 (2014): s5–s13. https://doi.org /10.2337/dc14-S005.

American Indian Center of Chicago. "Mission Statement." Accessed December 20, 2020. https://aicchicago.org/mission-statement/.

———. "Statement on Blackhawks." Accessed July 11, 2019. https://www.aicchicago.org /statement-on-blackhawks.

Arends, Wade B., Jr. "A Socio-Cultural Study of the Relocated American Indians in Chicago." Master's thesis, University of Chicago, 1958.

Aretæus of Cappadocia. "On Diabetes." In *Diabetes: A Medical Odyssey*, 1–6. Tuckahoe NY: USV Pharmaceutical Corp, 1971.

Aretæus of Cappadocia, Francis Adams, and Sydenham Society. *The Extant Works of Aretaeus, the Cappadocian.* London: Printed for the Sydenham Society, 1856.

Arndt, Grant. "'Contrary to Our Way of Thinking': The Struggle for an American Indian Center in Chicago, 1946–1953." *American Indian Culture and Research Journal* 22, no. 4 (January 1998): 117–34. https://doi.org/10.17953/aicr.22.4.14708636402211h2.

———. "The Nation in the City." In Straus, *Native Chicago*, 337–41.

———. "Relocation's Imagined Landscape and the Rise of Chicago's Native American Community." In Straus, *Native Chicago*, 159–72.

Beck, David R. M. *The Chicago American Indian Community, 1893–1988: Annotated Bibliography and Guide to Sources in Chicago.* Chicago: NAES College Press, 1988.

———. "The Chicago American Indian Community: An 'Invisible' Minority." In *Beyond Black and White*, edited by Maxine Seller and Lois Weis, 45–60. Albany: State University of New York Press, 1997.

Becker, Gaylene. *Disrupted Lives: How People Create Meaning in a Chaotic World.* Berkeley: University of California Press, 1997.

Benedict, Ruth. "Anthropology and the Abnormal." *Journal of General Psychology* 10, no. 2 (1934): 59–82. https://doi.org/10.1080/00221309.1934.9917714.

Bennett, Robert L., Philleo Nash, Helen Peterson, Gerald One Feather, and LaDonna Harris. "Relocation." In *Indian Self-Rule: First-Hand Accounts of Indian-White Relations from Roosevelt to Reagan*, edited by Kenneth R. Philp, 161–73. Salt Lake City: Howe Brothers, 1986.

Benyshek, Daniel C. "The 'Early Life' Origins of Obesity-Related Health Disorders: New Discoveries Regarding the Intergenerational Transmission of Developmentally Programmed Traits in the Global Cardiometabolic Health Crisis." *American Journal of Physical Anthropology* 152, no. S57 (October 2013): 79–93. https://doi.org/10.1002/ajpa.22393.

Biolsi, Thomas. "The Birth of the Reservation: Making the Modern Individual among the Lakota." *American Ethnologist* 22, no. 1 (February 1995): 28–53. https://doi.org/10.1525/ae.1995.22.1.02a00020.

Birnbaum, Morris J. "Rejoinder: Genetic Research into the Causes of Type 2 Diabetes Mellitus." *Anthropology & Medicine* 12, no. 2 (2005): 129–34. https://doi.org/10.1080/13648470500139908.

Björntorp, Per. "Abdominal Obesity and the Development of Noninsulin-Dependent Diabetes Mellitus." *Diabetes/Metabolism Reviews* 4, no. 6 (September 1988): 615–22. https://doi.org/10.1002/dmr.5610040607.

———. "Body Fat Distribution, Insulin Resistance, and Metabolic Diseases." *Nutrition* 13, no. 9 (September 1997): 795–803. https://doi.org/10.1016/s0899-9007(97)00191-3.

———. "Do Stress Reactions Cause Abdominal Obesity and Comorbidities?" *Obesity Reviews* 2, no. 2 (July 2001): 73–86. https://doi.org/10.1046/j.1467-789x.2001.00027.x.

———. "Visceral Fat Accumulation: the Missing Link between Psychosocial Factors and Cardiovascular Disease?" *Journal of Internal Medicine* 230, no. 3 (September 1991): 195–201. https://doi.org/10.1111/j.1365-2796.1991.tb00431.x.

Blackhawk, Ned. "I Can Carry On from Here: The Relocation of American Indians to Los Angeles." *Wicazo Sa Review* 11, no. 2 (Autumn 1995): 16–30. https://doi.org /10.2307/1409093.

Bordo, Susan. *Unbearable Weight: Feminism, Western Culture, and the Body*. Berkeley: University of California Press, 1993.

Bourdieu, Pierre. "The Taste of Luxury, Taste of Necessity." In *The Taste Culture Reader: Experiencing Food and Drink*, edited by Carolyn Korsmeyer, 72–78. New York: Berg, 2005.

Bowker, Geoffrey C., and Susan Leigh Star. *Sorting Things Out: Classification and Its Consequences (Inside Technology)*. Cambridge: MIT Press, 1999.

Broom, Dorothy, and Andrea Whittaker. "Controlling Diabetes, Controlling Diabetics: Moral Language in the Management of Diabetes Type 2." *Social Science & Medicine* 58, no. 11 (June 2004): 2371–82. https://doi.org/10.1016/j.socscimed.2003.09.002.

Bruna, Sean. "Religious Gardens, Pilgrimages, and Dancing: A Critique of Translated Interventions in a Tribal Community." In *The Applied Anthropology of Obesity: Prevention, Intervention, and Identity*, edited by Chad T. Morris and Alexandra G. Lancey, 121–40. Lanham MD: Lexington Books, 2015.

Buchanan, Thomas A. "(How) Can We Prevent Type 2 Diabetes?" *Diabetes* 56, no. 6 (June 2007): 1502–7. https://doi.org/10.2337/db07-0140.

Burt, Larry W. *Tribalism in Crisis: Federal Indian Policy, 1953–1961*. Albuquerque: University of New Mexico Press, 1982.

Cantrell, Betty Geishirt. "Access and Barriers to Food Items and Food Preparation among Plains Indians." *Wicazo Sa Review* 16, no. 1 (Spring 2001): 65–74. https://doi.org /10.1353/wic.2001.0002.

Caplan, Pat. "Approaches to the Study of Food, Health, and Identity." In *Food, Health and Identity*, edited by Pat Caplan, 1–31. New York: Routledge, 1997.

Casazza, Krista, Lynac J. Hanks, T. Mark Beasley, and Jose R. Fernandez. "Beyond Thriftiness: Independent and Interactive Effects of Genetic and Dietary Factors on Variations in Fat Deposition and Distribution Across Populations." *American Journal of Physical Anthropology* 145, no. 2 (March 2011): 181–91. https://doi.org/10.1002 /ajpa.21483.

Cattelino, Jessica R. *High Stakes: Florida Seminole Gaming and Sovereignty*. Durham NC: Duke University Press, 2008.

Cave, Alfred A. "Abuse of Power: Andrew Jackson and the Indian Removal Act Of 1830." *Historian* 65, no. 6 (December 2003): 1330–53. https://doi.org/10.1111/j.0018-2370 .2003.00055.x.

Centers for Disease Control and Prevention. "2017 Diabetes Report Card." Atlanta: United States Department of Health and Human Services, 2017.

——— . "National Diabetes Statistics Report, 2020: Estimates of Diabetes and Its Burden in the United States." Atlanta: United States Department of Health and Human Services, 2020.

Chicago American Indian Oral History Pilot Project. 1982–1985. "Native Voices in the City." Chicago: Newberry Library. Ayer Modern MS Oral History, Box 1.

————. 1983–1985. Chicago American Indian Oral History Project. Records 1982–1985 Transcripts. Chicago: Newberry Library. Ayer Modern MS Oral History, Boxes 2–3.

Christopoulou-Aletra, H., and N. Papavramidou. "'Diabetes' as Described by Byzantine Writers from the Fourth to the Ninth Century AD: The Graeco-Roman Influence." *Diabetologia* 51, no. 5 (May 2008): 892–96. https://doi.org/10.1007/s00125-008-0981-4.

Clark, Blue. *Lone Wolf v. Hitchcock: Treaty Rights and Indian Law at the End of the Nineteenth Century.* Lincoln: University of Nebraska Press, 1994.

Clarke, Adele E., Janet K. Shim, Laura Mamo, Jennifer Ruth Fosket, and Jennifer R. Fishman. "Biomedicalization: Technoscientific Transformations of Health, Illness, and U.S. Biomedicine." *American Sociological Review* 68, no. 2 (April 2003): 161–94. https://doi.org/10.2307/1519765.

Clarke, S. F., and J. R. Foster. "A History of Blood Glucose Meters and Their Role in Self-Monitoring of Diabetes Mellitus." *British Journal of Biomedical Science* 69, no. 2 (2012): 83–93. https://doi.org/10.1080/09674845.2012.12002443.

Clifford, James. *The Predicament of Culture: Twentieth-Century Ethnography, Literature, and Art.* Cambridge MA: Harvard University Press, 1988.

Conklin, Harold C. "Hanunóo Color Categories." *Southwestern Journal of Anthropology* 11, no. 4 (Winter 1955): 339–44. https://doi.org/10.1086/soutjanth.11.4.3628909.

Connerton, Paul. *How Societies Remember.* Cambridge: Cambridge University Press, 1989.

Counihan, Carole. *The Anthropology of Food and Body: Gender, Meaning, and Power.* New York: Routledge, 1999.

Cowger, Thomas W. *The National Congress of American Indians: The Founding Years.* Lincoln: University of Nebraska Press, 1999.

Crapanzano, Vincent. *Tuhami, Portrait of a Moroccan.* Chicago: University of Chicago Press, 1980.

Crosby, Alfred W. "Virgin Soil Epidemics as a Factor in the Aboriginal Depopulation in America." *William and Mary Quarterly* 33, no. 2 (April 1976): 289–99. https://doi.org/10.2307/1922166.

de Cora, Lorelei. "The Diabetic Plague in Indian Country: Legacy of Displacement." *Wicazo Sa Review* 16, no. 1 (Spring 2001): 9–15. https://doi.org/10.1353/wic.2001.0005.

Deloria, Philip Joseph. *Indians in Unexpected Places.* Lawrence: University Press of Kansas, 2004.

Deloria, Vine, Jr. *Custer Died for Your Sins: An Indian Manifesto.* New York: Macmillan, 1969.

Deloria, Vine, Jr., and Clifford M. Lytle. *The Nations Within: The Past and Future of American Indian Sovereignty.* New York: Pantheon Books, 1984.

Dumit, Joseph. *Drugs for Life: How Pharmaceutical Companies Define Our Health.* Durham NC: Duke University Press, 2012.

Eagle, Adam (Nordwall) Fortunate. "Urban Indians and the Occupation of Alcatrz Island." In *American Indian Activism: Alcatraz to the Longest Walk,* edited by Troy Johnson, Joane Nagel, and Duane Champagne, 52–73. Urbana: University of Illinois Press, 1997.

Epstein, Steven. *Inclusion: The Politics of Difference in Medical Research*. Chicago: University of Chicago Press, 2007.

Evaneshko, Veronica. "Presenting Complaints in a Navajo Indian Diabetic Population." In Joe and Young, *Diabetes as a Disease of Civilization*, 357–77.

Fagot-Campagna, Anne, K. M. Venkat Narayan, and Giuseppina Imperatore. "Type 2 Diabetes in Children." *British Medical Journal* 322, no. 7283 (February 2001): 377–78. https://doi.org/10.1136/bmj.322.7283.377.

Farmer, Paul. *Infections and Inequalities: The Modern Plagues*. Berkeley: University of California Press, 2001.

———. "On Suffering and Structural Violence: A View from Below." *Daedalus* 125, no. 1 (Winter 1996): 261–83.

———. *Pathologies of Power: Health, Human Rights, and the New War on the Poor*. Berkeley: University of California Press, 2003.

Ferreira, Mariana K. Leal, and Gretchen Chesley Lang. *Indigenous Peoples and Diabetes: Community Empowerment and Wellness*. Durham NC: Carolina Academic Press, 2006.

———. "Introduction: Deconstructing Diabetes." In Ferreira and Lang, *Indigenous Peoples and Diabetes*, 3–32.

Ferzacca, Steve. "'Actually, I Don't Feel That Bad': Managing Diabetes and the Clinical Encounter." *Medical Anthropology Quarterly* 14, no. 1 (March 2000): 28–50. https://doi.org/10.1525/maq.2000.14.1.28.

———. *Healing the Modern in a Central Javanese City*. Durham NC: Carolina Academic Press, 2001.

Feudtner, Chris. "Diabetes." In *Encyclopedia of Disability*, edited by Gary L. Albrecht, Jerome Bickenbach, David T. Mitchell, Walton O. Schalick, and Sharon L. Snyder, 397–99. Thousand Oaks CA: Sage Publications, 2006.

Fine, Ben. "Towards a Political Economy of Food." *Review of International Political Economy* 1, no. 3 (Autumn 1994): 519–45. https://doi.org/10.1080/09692299408434297.

Firth, Raymond. "Twins, Birds and Vegetables: Problems of Identification in Primitive Religious Thought." *Man* 1, no. 1 (March 1966): 1–17. https://doi.org/10.2307/2795897.

Fixico, Donald Lee. *Termination and Relocation: Federal Indian Policy, 1945–1960*. Albuquerque: University of New Mexico Press, 1986.

Forbes, Jack. "The Urban Tradition among Native Americans." *American Indian Culture and Research Journal* 22, no. 4 (1998): 15–41. https://doi.org/10.17953/aicr.22.4.e5m62705k64811k4.

Foucault, Michel. *Discipline and Punish: The Birth of the Prison*. New York: Vintage Books, 1995.

Frake, Charles O. "The Diagnosis of Disease among the Subanun of Mindanao." *American Anthropologist* 63, no. 1 (February 1961): 113–32. https://doi.org/10.1525/aa.1961.63.1.02a00070.

Fretts, Amanda M., Barbara V. Howard, Andrea M. Kriska, Nicolas L. Smith, Thomas Lumley, Elisa T. Lee, Marie Russell, and David Siscovick. "Physical Activity and Incident Diabetes in American Indians: The Strong Heart Study." *American Journal of Epidemiology* 170, no. 5 (September 2009): 632–39. https://doi.org/10.1093/aje/kwp181.

Fullwiley, Duana. *The Enculturated Gene: Sickle Cell Health Politics and Biological Difference in West Africa*. Princeton: Princeton University Press, 2011.

Galen. *Galen on Diseases and Symptoms*. Translated by Ian Johnston. Cambridge: Cambridge University Press, 2006.

Gallo, Mia V., and Lawrence M. Schell. "Height, Weight, and Body Mass Index among Akwesasne Mohawk Youth." *American Journal of Human Biology* 17, no. 3 (May 2005): 269–79. https://doi.org/10.1002/ajhb.20316.

Galtung, Johan. "Violence, Peace, and Peace Research." *Journal of Peace Research* 6, no. 3 (September 1969): 167–91. https://doi.org/10.1177/002234336900600301.

Garbarino, Merwyn S. "Life in the City: Chicago." In *The American Indian in Urban Society*, edited by Jack O. Waddell and O. Michael Watson, 168–205. New York: University Press of America, 1984.

Garcia, Orlando. "Urbanization of Rural Population: An American Indian Perspective." In Straus, *Native Chicago*, 193–204.

Garcia-Smith, Dianna. "The Gila River Diabetes Prevention Model." In Joe and Young, *Diabetes as a Disease of Civilization*, 471–94.

Garro, Linda C. "Intracultural Variation in Causal Accounts of Diabetes: A Comparison of Three Canadian Anishinaabe (Ojibway) Communities." *Culture, Medicine & Psychiatry* 20, no. 4 (December 1996): 381–420. https://doi.org/10.1007/BF00117086.

———. "Remembering What One Knows and the Construction of the Past: A Comparison of Cultural Consensus Theory and Cultural Schema Theory." *Ethos* 28, no. 3 (September 2000): 275–319. https://doi.org/10.1525/eth.2000.28.3.275.

Garro, Linda C., and Gretchen Chesley Lang. "Explanations of Diabetes: Anishinaabeg and Dakota Deliberate upon a New Illness." In Joe and Young, *Diabetes as a Disease of Civilization*, 293–328.

Garroutte, Eva Marie. "The Racial Formation of American Indians: Negotiating Legitimate Identities within Tribal and Federal Law." *American Indian Quarterly* 25, no. 2 (Spring 2001): 224–39. https://doi.org/10.1353/aiq.2001.0020.

Gemmill, C. L. "The Greek Concept of Diabetes." *Bulletin of the New York Academy of Medicine* 48, no. 8 (September 1972): 1033–36.

George, Kenneth M. *Picturing Islam: Art and Ethics in a Muslim Lifeworld*. Chichester: John Wiley & Sons, 2011.

Gilliland, Frank D., Charles Owen, Susan S. Gilliland, and Janette S. Carter. "Temporal Trends in Diabetes Mortality among American Indians and Hispanics in New Mexico: Birth Cohort and Period Effects." *American Journal of Epidemiology* 145, no. 5 (March 1997): 422–31. https://doi.org/10.1093/oxfordjournals.aje.a009124.

Gohdes, D. M. "Diabetes in American Indians: A Growing Problem." *Diabetes Care* 9, no. 6 (November 1986): 609–13. https://doi.org/10.2337/diacare.9.6.609.

Goldberg-Ambrose, Carole. "Of Native Americans and Tribal Members: The Impact of Law on Indian Group Life." *Law & Society Review* 28, no. 5 (1994): 1123–48. https://doi.org/10.2307/3054025.

Gonzales, Angela. "The (Re)Articulation of American Indian Identity: Maintaining Boundaries and Regulating Access to Ethnically Tied Resources." *American Indian Culture and Research Journal* 22, no. 4 (January 1998): 199–225. https://doi.org/10.17953/aicr.22.4.3766063k674q4808.

Grinker, Roy. 2007. *Unstrange Minds: Remapping the World of Autism*. Philadelphia: Basic Books, 2007.

Grinnell, George Bird. *The Cheyenne Indians: Their History and Ways of Life*. Vol. 1. Lincoln: University of Nebraska Press, 1972.

Guell, Cornelia. "Self-Care at the Margins: Meals and Meters in Migrants' Diabetes Tactics." *Medical Anthropology Quarterly* 26, no. 4 (December 2012): 518–33. https://doi.org/10.1111/maq.12005.

Guss, David M. "Cimarrones, Theater, and the State." In *History, Power, and Identity: Ethnogenesis in the Americas, 1492–1992*, edited by Jonathan Hill, 180–92. Iowa City: University of Iowa Press, 1996.

———. "The Selling of San Juan: The Performance of History in an Afro-Venezuelan Community." *American Ethnologist* 20, no. 3 (August 1993): 451–73. https://doi.org/10.1525/ae.1993.20.3.02a00010.

Hacking, Ian. "Making Up People." In *Beyond the Body Proper: Reading the Anthropology of Material Life*, edited by Margaret M. Lock and Judith Farquhar, 150–63. Durham NC: Duke University Press, 2007.

Hales, C. N., and D. J. P. Barker. 1992. "Type 2 (Non-Insulin-Dependent) Diabetes Mellitus: The Thrifty Phenotype Hypothesis." *Diabetologia* 35, no.7 (July 1992): 595–601. https://doi.org/10.1007/BF00400248.

Hamilton, Marc T., Deborah G. Hamilton, and Theodore W. Zderic. "Role of Low Energy Expenditure and Sitting in Obesity, Metabolic Syndrome, Type 2 Diabetes, and Cardiovascular Disease." *Diabetes* 56, no. 11 (November 2007): 2655–67. https://doi.org/10.2337/db07-0882.

Harmon, Alexandra. "Tribal Enrollment Councils: Lessons on Law and Indian Identity." *Western Historical Quarterly* 32, no. 2 (Summer 2001): 175–200. https://doi.org/10.2307/3650772.

Hartmann, William E., and Joseph P. Gone. "American Indian Historical Trauma: Community Perspectives from Two Great Plains Medicine Men." *American Journal of Community Psychology* 54, nos. 3–4 (December 2014): 274–88. https://doi.org/10.1007/s10464-014-9671-1.Hearst, M. O., N. Laska M, J. H. Himes, M. Butterbrodt, A. Sinaiko, R. Iron Cloud, M. Tobacco, and M. Story. 2011. "The Co-Occurrence of Obesity, Elevated Blood Pressure, and Acanthosis Nigricans among American Indian School Children: Identifying Individual Heritage and Environment-Level Correlates." *American Journal of Human Biology* 23, no. 3 (May/June 2011): 346–52. https://doi.org/10.1002/ajhb.21140.

Heinemann, Laura Lynn. "For the Sake of Others: Reciprocal Webs of Obligation and the Pursuit of Transplantation as a Caring Act." *Medical Anthropology Quarterly* 28, no. 1 (March 2014): 66–84. https://doi.org/10.1111/maq.12060.

Henschen, Folke. "On the Term Diabetes in the Works of Aretaeus and Galen." *Medical History* 13, no. 2 (April 1969): 190–92. https://doi.org/10.1017/s0025727300014277.

Herzfeld, Michael. *The Body Impolitic: Artisans and Artifice in the Global Hierarchy of Value*. Chicago: University of Chicago Press, 2004.

Hickey, Martin, and Janette Carter. "Cultural Barriers to Delivering Healthcare: The Non-Indian Provider Perspective." In Joe and Young, *Diabetes as a Disease of Civilization*, 453–70.

Hill, Jonathan, and Thomas Wilson. "Identity Politics and the Politics of Identities." *Identities: Global Studies in Culture and Power* 10, no. 1 (2003): 1–8. https://doi.org/10.1080/10702890304336.

Himsworth, H. P. "Diabetes Mellitus: Its Differentiation into Insulin-Sensitive and Insulin-Insensitive Types. 1936." *International Journal of Epidemiology* 42, no. 6 (December 2013): 1594–98. https://doi.org/10.1093/ije/dyt203.

House Concurrent Resolution 108, *U.S. Statutes at Large* 67 (1953).

Hrdlička, Aleš. *Physiological and Medical Observations among the Indians of Southwestern United States and Northern Mexico, Bulletin—Smithsonian Institution Bureau of American Ethnology* no. 34. Washington DC: U.S. Government Printing Office, 1908.

Hunleth, Jean. 2013. "Children's Roles in Tuberculosis Treatment Regimes: Constructing Childhood and Kinship in Urban Zambia." *Medical Anthropology Quarterly* 27 no. 2 (June 2013): 292–311. https://doi.org/10.1111/maq.12028.

Hunt, Linda M. "Moral Reasoning and the Meaning of Cancer: Causal Explanations of Oncologists and Patients in Southern Mexico." *Medical Anthropology Quarterly* 12, no. 3 (September 1998): 298–318. https://doi.org/10.1525/maq.1998.12.3.298.

Hunt, Linda M., and Nedal H. Arar. "An Analytical Framework for Contrasting Patient and Provider Views of the Process of Chronic Disease Management." *Medical Anthropology Quarterly* 15, no. 3 (September 2001): 347–67. https://doi.org/10.1525/maq.2001.15.3.347.

Indian Health Service. "Gold Book." Rockville MD: U.S. Department of Health and Human Services, 2007.

Intertribal Friendship House, Community History Project, and Susan Lobo. *Urban Voices: The Bay Area American Indian Community*. Tucson: University of Arizona Press, 2002.

Iverson, Peter. "Knowing the Land, Leaving the Land: Navajos, Hopis, and Relocation in the American West." *Montana: The Magazine of Western History* 38, no. 1 (1988): 67–70.

——— . *"We Are Still Here:" American Indians in the Twentieth Century*. Wheeling IL: Harlan Davidson, 1998.

Iverson, Peter, and Monty Roessel. *Diné: A History of the Navajos*. Albuquerque: University of New Mexico Press, 2002.

Jackson, Deborah Davis. *Our Elders Lived It: American Indian Identity in the City*. DeKalb: Northern Illinois University Press, 2002.

——— . "This Hole in Our Heart: Urban Indian Identity and the Power of Silence." *American Indian Culture and Research Journal* 22, no. 4 (1998): 227–54. https://doi.org/10.17953/aicr.22.4.u255428317312708.

————. "A Place Where I Can Let My Hair Down: From Social Club to Cultural Center in an Urban Indian Community." *City & Society* 13, no. 1 (June 2001): 31–55. https://doi.org/10.1525/city.2001.13.1.31.

Jackson, M. Yvonne. "Diet, Culture, and Diabetes." In Joe and Young, *Diabetes as a Disease of Civilization*, 381–406.

Jackson, Michael. *Minima Ethnographica: Intersubjectivity and the Anthropological Project*. Chicago: University of Chicago Press, 1998.

Jaeger, Lisa, David Raasch, Igor Sopronenko, and Jimmy Fall. *Tribal Nations: The Story of Federal Indian Law*, 2006.

Jarding, Lilias Jones. "Tribal-State Relations Involving Land and Resources in the Self-Determination Era." *Political Research Quarterly* 57, no. 2 (June 2004): 295–303. https://doi.org/10.2307/3219872.

Joe, Jennie Rose, and Robert S. Young, eds. *Diabetes as a Disease of Civilization: The Impact of Culture Change on Indigenous Peoples*. Berlin: Mouton de Gruyter, 1993.

Jones, David S. "Death, Uncertainty, and Rhetoric." In *Beyond Germs*, edited by Catherine M. Cameron, Paul Kelton, and Alan C. Swedlund, 16–49. Tucson: University of Arizona Press, 2015.

Joslin, Elliott P. "The Universality of Diabetes: A Survey of Diabetic Morbidity in Arizona." *Journal of the American Medical Association* 115, no. 24 (1940): 2033–38. https://doi.org/doi:10.1001/jama.1940.02810500001001.

Justice, James. "The History of Diabetes in the Desert People." In Joe and Young, *Diabetes as a Disease of Civilization*, 69–128.

Kiesling, Scott Fabius. "'Now I Gotta Watch What I Say': Shifting Constructions of Masculinity in Discourse." *Journal of Linguistic Anthropology* 11, no. 2 (December 2001): 250–73. https://doi.org/10.1525/jlin.2001.11.2.250.

King, Cecil. "Here Come the Anthros." In *Ethnographic Fieldwork: An Anthropological Reader*, edited by Antonius C. G. M. Robben and Jeffrey A. Sluka, 191–93. Malden MA: Blackwell, 2007.

King, Patricia J. "Urbanization and the Evolution of Modern American Indian Tribalism, Los Angeles and San Francisco, 1950–1970." Master's thesis, Northern Arizona University, 2006.

Klawiter, Maren. "Regulatory Shifts, Pharmaceutical Scripts, and the New Consumption Junction: Configuring High-Risk, Women in an Era of Chemoprevention." In *The New Political Sociology of Science: Institutions, Networks, and Power*, edited by Scott Frickel and Kelly Moore, 432–60. Madison: University of Wisconsin Press, 2006.

Knorr Cetina, Karin. *Epistemic Cultures: How the Sciences Make Knowledge*. Cambridge MA: Harvard University Press, 1999.

Knowler, William C., David J. Pettitt, Peter H. Bennett, and Robert C. Williams. "Diabetes Mellitus in the Pima Indians: Genetic and Evolutionary Considerations." *American Journal of Physical Anthropology* 62, no. 1 (September 1983): 107–14. https://doi.org/10.1002/ajpa.1330620114.

Knowler, William C., David J. Pettitt, Mohammed F. Saad, and Peter H. Bennett. "Diabetes Mellitus in the Pima Indians: Incidence, Risk Factors and Pathogenesis." *Diabetes/Metabolism Reviews* 6, no. 1 (February 1990): 1–27. https://doi.org/10.1002/dmr.5610060101.

Knowler, William C., David J. Pettitt, Peter J. Savage, and Peter H. Bennett. 1981. "Diabetes Incidence in Pima Indians: Contributions of Obesity and Parental Diabetes." *American Journal of Epidemiology* no. 113, no. 2 (February 1981): 144–56. https://doi.org/10.1093/oxfordjournals.aje.a113079.

Kramer, B. J. "Health and Aging of Urban American Indians." *Western Journal of Medicine* 157, no. 3 (September 1992): 281–85.

Kreiner, Meta J., and Linda M. Hunt. "The Pursuit of Preventive Care for Chronic Illness: Turning Healthy People into Chronic Patients." *Sociology of Health & Illness* 36, no. 6 (July 2014): 870–84. https://doi.org/10.1111/1467-9566.12115.

Kriska, Andrea M., Aramesh Saremi, Robert L. Hanson, Peter H. Bennett, Sayuko Kobes, Desmond E. Williams, and William C. Knowler. "Physical Activity, Obesity, and the Incidence of Type 2 Diabetes in a High-Risk Population." *American Journal of Epidemiology* 158 no. 7 (2003): 669–75. https://doi.org/10.1093/aje/kwg191.

Krouse, Susan Applegate. "Traditional Iroquois Socials: Maintaining Identity in the City." *American Indian Quarterly* 25, no. 3 (Summer 2001): 400–408. https://doi.org/10.1353/aiq.2001.0049.

LaGrand, James B. *Indian Metropolis: Native Americans in Chicago, 1945–75*. Urbana: University of Illinois Press, 2002.

———. "Indian Work and Indian Neighborhoods: Adjusting to Life in Chicago during the 1950s." In *Enduring Nations: Native Americans in the Midwest*, edited by R. David Edmunds, 195–213. Urbana: University of Illinois Press, 2008.

Lajimodiere, Denise. "A Healing Journey." *Wicazo Sa Review* 27, no. 2 (Fall 2012): 5–19. https://doi.org/10.5749/wicazosareview.27.2.0005.

Lang, Gretchen Chesley. "'In Their Tellings': Dakota Narratives about History and the Body." In Ferreira and Lang, *Indigenous Peoples and Diabetes*, 53–71.

———. "Talking about a New Illness with the Dakota: Reflections on Diabetes, Foods and Culture." In Ferreira and Lang, *Indigenous Peoples and Diabetes*, 203–30.

Lapier, Rosalyn, and David R. M. Beck. "A 'One-Man Relocation Team': Scott Henry Peters and American Indian Urban Migration in the 1930s." *Western Historical Quarterly* 45, no. 1 (Spring 2014): 17–36. https://doi.org/10.2307/westhistquar.45.1.0017.

Latour, Bruno, and Steve Woolgar. *Laboratory Life: The Construction of Scientific Facts.* Princeton: Princeton University Press, 1986.

Lazewski, Tony. "American Indian Migration to and within Chicago, Illinois." PhD diss., University of Illinois, 1976.

Levinson, David. "An Explanation for the Oneida-Colonist Alliance in the American Revolution." *Ethnohistory* 23, no. 3 (Summer 1976): 265–89. https://doi.org/10.2307/481255.

Lewis, David Rich. "Still Native: The Significance of Native Americans in the History of the Twentieth-Century American West." *Western Historical Quarterly* 24 no. 2 (May 1993): 203–27. https://doi.org/10.2307/970936.

Livingston, Julie. *Improvising Medicine: An African Oncology Ward in an Emerging Cancer Epidemic*. Durham NC: Duke University Press, 2012.

Lobo, Susan. "Is Urban a Person or a Place? Characteristics of Urban Indian Country." *American Indian Culture and Research Journal* 22, no. 4 (1998): 89–102. https://doi .org/10.17953/aicr.22.4.y12173126u68786t.

Lock, Margaret M. *Twice Dead: Organ Transplants and the Reinvention of Death*. Berkeley: University of California Press, 2002.

Lock, Margaret M., and Vinh-Kim Nguyen. *An Anthropology of Biomedicine*. Malden MA: Wiley-Blackwell, 2010.

Lomawaima, K. Tsianina. "Domesticity in the Federal Indian Schools: The Power of Authority over Mind and Body." *American Ethnologist* 20, no. 2 (May 1993): 227–40. https://doi.org/10.1525/ae.1993.20.2.02a00010.

Low, John N. *Imprints: The Pokagon Band of Potawatomi Indians and the City of Chicago*. East Lansing: Michigan State University Press, 2016.

Macaulay, Ann C., Treena Delormier, Alex M. McComber, Edward J. Cross, Louise P. Potvin, Gilles Paradis, Rhonda L. Kirby, Chantal Saad-Haddad, and Serge Desrosiers. "Participatory Research with Native Community of Kahnawake Creates Innovative Code of Research Ethics." *Canadian Journal of Public Health* 89, no. 2 (1998): 105–8. https://doi.org/10.1007/BF03404399.

Martin, Emily. "The Woman in the Flexible Body." In *Revisioning Women, Health and Healing: Feminist, Cultural, and Technoscience Perspectives*, edited by Adele Clarke and Virginia L. Olesen, 97–115. New York: Routledge, 1999.

Matthews, Steven G., and David I. W. Phillips. "Minireview: Transgenerational Inheritance of the Stress Response: A New Frontier in Stress Research." *Endocrinology* 151, no. 1 (January 2010): 7–13. https://doi.org/10.1210/en.2009-0916.

Maybury-Lewis, David. *Indigenous Peoples, Ethnic Groups, and the State*. Boston: Allyn and Bacon, 1997.

McCarthy, Robert. "The Bureau of Indian Affairs and the Federal Trust Obligation to American Indians." *Brigham Young University Journal of Public Law* no. 19, no. 1 (2004): 1–160.

McCombie, Susan C. "Folk Flu and Viral Syndrome: An Anthropological Perspective." In *Anthropology in Public Health: Bridging Differences in Culture and Society*, edited by Robert A. Hahn, 27–43. Oxford: Oxford University Press, 1999.

Mendenhall, Emily, Rebecca A. Seligman, Alicia Fernandez, and Elizabeth A. Jacobs. "Speaking through Diabetes." *Medical Anthropology Quarterly* 24, no. 2 (June 2010): 220–39. https://doi.org/10.1111/j.1548-1387.2010.01098.x.

Meriam, Lewis, and Hubert Work. *The Problem of Indian Administration: Report of a Survey Made at the Request of Honorable Hubert Work, Secretary of the Interior, and Submitted to Him, February 21, 1928*. Baltimore: Johns Hopkins Press, 1928.

Meyer, Melissa L. "American Indian Blood Quantum Requirements: Blood Is Thicker Than Family." In *Over the Edge: Remapping the American West*, edited by Valerie J. Matsumoto and Blake Allmendinger, 231–49. Berkeley: University of California Press, 1999.

Mihesuah, Devon A. "Decolonizing Our Diets by Recovering Our Ancestors' Gardens." *American Indian Quarterly* 27, nos. 3–4 (Summer–Fall 2003): 807–39. https://doi .org/10.1353/aiq.2004.0084.

——. *Recovering Our Ancestors' Gardens: Indigenous Recipes and Guide to Diet and Fitness*. Rev. ed. Lincoln: University of Nebraska Press, 2020.

——. *So You Want to Write about American Indians? A Guide for Writers, Students, and Scholars*. Lincoln: University of Nebraska Press, 2005.

Miller, Douglas K. *Indians on the Move*. Chapel Hill: University of North Carolina Press, 2019.

——. "Willing Workers: Urban Relocation and American Indian Initiative, 1940s–1960s." *Ethnohistory* 60, no. 1 (Winter 2013): 51–76. https://doi.org/10.1215/00141801 -1816175.

Mol, Annemarie. *The Body Multiple: Ontology in Medical Practice*. Durham NC: Duke University Press, 2002.

——. *The Logic of Care: Health and the Problem of Patient Choice*. New York: Routledge, 2008.

——. "What Diagnostic Devices Do: The Case of Blood Sugar Measurement." *Theoretical Medicine and Bioethics* 21, no. 1 (January 2000): 9–22. https://doi.org/10 .1023/a:1009999119586.

Morgan, William. *Diabetes Mellitus: Its History, Chemistry, Anatomy, Pathology, Physiology, and Treatment. Illustrated with Woodcuts, and Cases Successfully Treated*. London: Homeopathic Publishing Company, 1877.

Nagel, Joane. "American Indian Ethnic Renewal: Politics and the Resurgence of Identity." *American Sociological Review* 60, no. 6 (December 1995): 947–65. https://doi .org/10.2307/2096434.

Neel, James V. "Diabetes Mellitus: A 'Thrifty' Genotype Rendered Detrimental by 'Progress'?" *American Journal of Human Genetics* 14, no. 4 (December 1962): 353–62.

——. "The 'Thrifty Genotype' in 1998." *Nutrition Reviews* 57, no. 5 (May 1999): 2–9. https://doi.org/10.1111/j.1753-4887.1999.tb01782.x.

——. "The Thrifty Genotype Revisited." In *The Genetics of Diabetes Mellitus*, edited by J. Köbberling and R. Tattersall, 283–93. New York: Academic Press, 1982.

Neils, Elaine M. "Reservation to City: Indian Migration and Federal Relocation." Research paper no. 131, University of Chicago, Chicago, 1971.

Niehoff, Arthur. "Discussion." *Anthropological Quarterly* 39, no. 3 (1966): 244–53. https:// doi.org/10.2307/3316808.

Norris, Tina, Paula L. Vines, and Elizabeth M. Hoeffel. "The American Indian and Alaska Native Population: 2010." In *2010 Census Briefs*. United States Census Bureau: U.S. Department of Commerce: Economics and Statistics Administration, 2012.

Olesen, Virginia L. 1989. "Caregiving, Ethical and Informal: Emerging Challenges in the Sociology of Health and Illness." *Journal of Health and Social Behavior* 30, no. 1 (March 1989): 1–10. https://doi.org/10.2307/2136906.

Olson, Brooke. "Applying Medical Anthropology: Developing Diabetes Education and Prevention Programs in American Indian Cultures." *American Indian Culture and Research Journal* 23, no. 3 (1999): 185–203. https://doi.org/10.17953/aicr.23.3 .t01j41m05n4752p8.

———. "Meeting the Challenges of American Indian Diabetes: Anthropological Perspectives on Prevention and Treatment." In Trafzer and Weiner, *Medicine Ways*, 163–84.

Ono, Azusa. "I Am a Denver Indian: The Bureau of Indian Affairs' Relocation Program and Denver's Native American Community." In *Denver Inside and Out*, edited by Larry Borowsky, Jeanne E. Abrams, and History Colorado, 83–91. Denver: Colorado Historical Society, 2011.

Oritz, Lisa. "Indian or Not?" In Straus, *Native Chicago*, 437–42.

Ozanne, S. E., and C. N. Hales. 1998. "Thrifty Yes, Genetic No." *Diabetologia* 41, no. 4 (March 1998): 485–87. https://doi.org/10.1007/s001250050934.

Papaspyros, N. S. *The History of Diabetes Mellitus*. 2nd ed. Stuttgart: G. Thieme, 1964.

Paredes, J. Anthony. "Toward a Reconceptualization of American Indian Urbanization: A Chippewa Case." *Anthropological Quarterly* 44, no. 4 (October 1971): 256–71. https://doi.org/10.2307/3316972.

Park, Peter. "What Is Participatory Research? A Theoretical and Methodological Perspective." In *Voices of Change: Participatory Research in the United States and Canada*, edited by P. Park, M. Brydon-Miller, B. Hall, and T. Jackson, 1–19. Westport CT: Bergin & Garvey, 1993.

Parker, Myra. "CBPR Principles and Research Ethics in Indian Country." In *Community-Based Participatry Resarch for Health: Advancing Social and Health Equity 3rd edition*, edited by Nina Wallerstein, Bonnie Duran, John G. Oetzel, and Meredith Minkler, 207–14. San Francisco: Jossey Bass, 2018.

Parry, Jane. 2010. "Pacific Islanders Pay Heavy Price for Abandoning Traditional Diet." *Bulletin of the World Health Organization* 88, no. 7 (2010): 484–85. https://doi.org /10.2471/BLT.10.010710.

Pavkov, Meda E., Robert L. Hanson, William C. Knowler, Peter H. Bennett, Jonathan Krakoff, and Robert G. Nelson. "Changing Patterns of Type 2 Diabetes Incidence among Pima Indians." *Diabetes Care* 30, no. 7 (July 2007): 1758–63. https://doi.org /10.2337/dc06-2010.

Pearson, J. Diane. "Lewis Cass and the Politics of Disease: The Indian Vaccination Act of 1832." *Wicazo Sa Review* 18, no. 2 (2003): 9–35. https://doi.org/10.1353/wic .2003.0017.

Petersen, Alan R., and Deborah Lupton. *The New Public Health: Health and Self in the Age of Risk*. London: Sage Publications, 1996.

Pettitt, David J., Jeffrey R. Lisse, William C. Knowler, and Peter H. Bennett. "Mortality as a Function of Obesity and Diabetes Mellitus." *American Journal of*

Epidemiology 115, no. 3 (March 1982): 359–66. https://doi.org/10.1093/oxford-journals.aje.a113313.

Philp, Kenneth R. "Stride toward Freedom: The Relocation of Indians to Cities, 1952–1960." *Western Historical Quarterly* 16, no. 2 (April 1985): 175–90. https://doi.org/10.2307/969660.

Pickering, Andrew. *The Mangle of Practice: Time, Agency, and Science*. Chicago: University of Chicago Press, 1995.

Pickup, J. C., and M. A. Crook. "Is Type II Diabetes Mellitus a Disease of the Innate Immune System?" *Diabetologia* 41, no. 10 (September 1998): 1241–48. https://doi.org/10.1007/s001250051058.

Poss, Jane, and Mary Ann Jezewski. "The Role and Meaning of *Susto* in Mexican Americans: Explanatory Model of Type 2 Diabetes." *Medical Anthropology Quarterly* 16, no. 3 (September 2002): 360–77. https://doi.org/10.1525/maq.2002.16.3.360.

Potvin, Louise, Margaret Cargo, Alex M. McComber, Treena Delormier, and Ann C. Macaulay. "Implementing Participatory Intervention and Research in Communities: Lessons from the Kahnawake Schools Diabetes Prevention Project in Canada." *Social Science & Medicine* 56, no. 6 (2003): 1295–305. https://doi.org/10.1016/S0277-9536(02)00129-6.

Ramirez, Renya K. *Native Hubs: Culture, Community, and Belonging in Silicon Valley and Beyond*. Durham NC: Duke University Press, 2007.

Rand, Katherine, and Steven Light. "Do 'Fish and Chips' Mix? The Politics of Indian Gaming in Wisconsin." *Gaming Law Review* 2, no. 2 (March 1998): 129–42. https://doi.org/10.1089/glr.1998.2.129.

Rapp, Rayna. "Real-Time Fetus." In *Cyborgs & Citadels: Anthropological Interventions in Emerging Sciences and Technologies*, edited by Gary Lee Downey and Joseph Dumit, 31–48. Santa Fe NM: School of American Research Press, 1997.

Rhoades, Dorothy A., Yvette Roubideaux, and Dedra Buchwald. "Diabetes Care among Older Urban American Indians and Alaska Natives." *Ethnicity and Disease* 14, no. 4 (Autumn 2004): 574–79.

Ricciardelli, Alex F. "The Adoption of White Agriculture by the Oneida Indians." *Ethnohistory* 10, no. 4 (Autumn 1963): 309–28. https://doi.org/10.2307/480333.

Rith-Najarian, R. J., S. E. Valway, and D. M. Ghodes. "Diabetes in a Northern Minnesota Chippewa Tribe: Prevalence and Incidence of Diabetes and Incidence of Major Complications, 1986–1988." *Diabetes Care* 16, no. 1 (January 1993): 266–70. https://doi.org/10.2337/diacare.16.1.266.

Ritzenthaler, Robert E. "The Oneida Indians of Wisconsin." *Bulletin of the Public Museum of the City of Milwaukee* 19, no. 1 (November 1950): 1–52.

Rock, Melanie. "Sweet Blood and Social Suffering: Rethinking Cause-Effect Relationships in Diabetes, Distress and Duress." *Medical Anthropology* 22, no. 2 (2003): 131–74. https://doi.org/10.1080/01459740306764.

Rosaldo, Michelle Zimbalist. "Metaphors and Folk Classification." *Southwestern Journal of Anthropology* 28, no. 1 (Spring 1972): 83–99. https://doi.org/10.1086/soutjanth.28.1.3629445.

Rose, Nikolas. "The Human Sciences in a Biological Age." *Theory, Culture & Society* 30, no. 1 (January 2013): 3–34. https://doi.org/10.1177/0263276412456569.

———. *The Politics of Life Itself: Biomedicine, Power, and Subjectivity in the Twenty-First Century.* Princeton: Princeton University Press, 2007.

Rosenfeld, Louis. "Insulin: Discovery and Controversy." *Clinical Chemistry* 48, no. 12 (December 2002): 2270–88. https://doi.org/10.1093/clinchem/48.12.2270.

Rosenthal, Nicolas G. *Reimagining Indian Country: Native American Migration & Identity in Twentieth-Century Los Angeles.* Chapel Hill: University of North Carolina Press, 2012.

Roy, Bernard. "Diabetes and Identity: Changes in the Food Habits of the Innu—A Critical Look at Health Professionals' Interventions Regarding Diet." In Ferreira and Lang, *Indigenous Peoples and Diabetes,* 167–86.

Sahota, Puneet Chawla. "Genetic Histories: Native Americans' Accounts of Being at Risk for Diabetes." *Social Studies of Science* no. 42, no. 6 (December 2012): 821–42. https://doi.org/10.1177/0306312712454044.

Sanders, Lee J. "From Thebes to Toronto and the 21st Century: An Incredible Journey." *Diabetes Spectrum* 15, no. 1 (January 2002): 56–60. https://doi.org/10.2337/diaspect.15.1.56.

Scheder, Jo C. "A Sickly-Sweet Harvest: Farmworker Diabetes and Social Equality." *Medical Anthropology Quarterly* 2, no. 3 (September 1988): 251–77. https://doi.org/10.1525/maq.1988.2.3.02a00050.

Scheper-Hughes, Nancy. "Forward: Diabetes and Genocide—Beyond the Thrifty Gene." In Ferreira and Lang, *Indigenous Peoples and Diabetes,* xvii–xxi.

Scheper-Hughes, Nancy, and Margaret M. Lock. "The Mindful Body: A Prolegomenon to Future Work in Medical Anthropology." *Medical Anthropology Quarterly* 1, no. 1 (March 1987): 6–41. https://doi.org/10.1525/maq.1987.1.1.02a00020.

Schneider, T. "Diabetes through the Ages: A Salute to Insulin." *South African Medical Journal* 46, no. 38 (September 1972): 1394–400.

Schoenberg, Nancy E., Elaine M. Drew, Eleanor Palo Stoller, and Cary S. Kart. "Situating Stress: Lessons from Lay Discourse on Diabetes." In *Anthropology and Public Health: Bridging Differences in Culture and Society,* edited by Robert A. Hahn and Marcia Claire Inhorn, 94–113. Oxford: Oxford University Press, 2009.

Schulz, Leslie O. "Traditional Environment Protects against Diabetes in Pima Indians." *Healthy Weight Journal* 13, no. 5 (1999): 68–70.

Schutz, Alfred. *Collected Papers I: The Problem of Social Reality.* The Hague: Martinus Nijhoff Publishers, 1962.

———. *On Phenomenology and Social Relations: Selected Writings.* Chicago: University of Chicago Press, 1970.

Seligman, Rebecca, Emily Mendenhall, Maria D. Valdovinos, Alicia Fernandez, and Elizabeth A. Jacobs. "Self-Care and Subjectivity among Mexican Diabetes Patients in the United States." *Medical Anthropology Quarterly* 29, no. 1 (March 2015): 61–79. https://doi.org/10.1111/maq.12107.

The Sigma Type Diabetes Consortium. "Sequence Variants in SLC16A11 Are a Common Risk Factor for Type 2 Diabetes in Mexico." *Nature* 506, no. 7486 (2014): 97–101. https://doi.org/10.1038/nature12828.

Simon, Scott. "Contesting Formosa: Tragic Remembrance, Urban Space, and National Identity in Taipak." *Identities: Global Studies in Culture and Power* 10, no. 1 (2003): 109–31. https://doi.org/10.1080/10702890304338.

Skinner, Michael K., Mohan Manikkam, and Carlos Guerrero-Bosagna. "Epigenetic Transgenerational Actions of Environmental Factors in Disease Etiology." *Trends in Endocrinology & Metabolism* 21, no. 4 (January 2010): 214–22. https://doi.org/10.1016/j.tem.2009.12.007.

Smith, Linda Tuhiwai. *Decolonizing Methodologies: Research and Indigenous Peoples.* London: Zed Books, 1999.

Smith-Morris, Carolyn. "Bhabha in the Clinic: Hybridity, Difference, and Decolonizing Health." *Medicine Anthropology Theory* 7, no. 2 (September 2020): 33–57. https://doi.org/10.17157/mat.7.2.687.

———. "'Community Participation' in Tribal Diabetes Programs." *American Indian Culture and Research Journal* 30, no. 2 (2006): 85–110. https://doi.org/10.17953/aicr.30.2.8g365u624u783550.

———. "Diagnostic Controversy: Gestational Diabetes and the Meaning of Risk for Pima Indian Women." *Medical Anthropology* 24 (2005): 145–77. https://doi.org/10.1080/01459740590933902.

Snipp, C. Matthew. "Sociological Perspectives on American Indians." *Annual Review of Sociology* 18 (August 1992): 351–71. https://doi.org/10.1146/annurev.so.18.080192.002031.

Snyder, Peter Z. "Kinship, Friendship, and Enclave: The Problem of American Indian Urbanization." In *American Indian Urbanization*, edited by Jack O. Waddell and O. Michael Watson, 117–29. West Lafayette IN: Purdue Research Foundation, 1973.

Sorkin, Alan L. *American Indians and Federal Aid*. Washington DC: Brookings Institution, 1971.

———. *The Urban American Indian.* Lexington MA: Lexington Books, 1978.

Southall, Aidan W. "The Illusion of Tribe." In *The Passing of Tribal Man in Africa*, edited by Peter C. W. Gutkind, 28–50. Leiden: E. J. Brill, 1970.

Southam, L., N. Soranzo, S. Montgomery, T. Frayling, M. McCarthy, I. Barroso, and E. Zeggini. "Is the Thrifty Genotype Hypothesis Supported by Evidence Based on Confirmed Type 2 Diabetes-and-Obesity-Susceptibility Variants?" *Diabetologia* 52, no. 9 (September 2009): 1846–51. https://doi.org/10.1007/s00125-009-1419-3.

Spanakis, Elias K., and Sherita Hill Golden. "Race/Ethnic Difference in Diabetes and Diabetic Complications." *Current Diabetes Reports* 13, no. 6 (September 2013): 814–23. https://doi.org/10.1007/s11892-013-0421-9.

Spicer, Edward H. "Indian Identity versus Assimilation." In *Occasional Papers of the Weatherhead Foundation*, 28–54. New York: Weatherhead Foundation, 1975.

St. Augustine's Center for American Indians. St. Augustine's Center for American Indians Records: 1966–1969 General Correspondence. Chicago: Newberry Library. Ayer Modern MS St. Augustine's, Box 5, 1961–2006.

Straus, Terry, ed. *Native Chicago*. Chicago: McNaughton and Gunn, 2002.

Straus, Terry, and Debra Valentino. "Retribalization in Urban Indian Communities." *American Indian Culture and Research Journal* 22, no. 4 (1998): 103–15. https://doi .org/10.17953/aicr.22.4.g4g7u036414w26m2.

Sturm, Circe. *Blood Politics: Race, Culture, and Identity in the Cherokee Nation of Oklahoma*. Berkeley: University of California Press, 2002.

Sutton, David. *Remembrance of Repasts: An Anthropology of Food and Memory*. Oxford: Berg, 2001.

Suzukovich, Eli, III. "The Seen and Unseen: Religion and Identity in the Chicago American Indian Community." PhD diss., University of Montana, 2011.

Szathmáry, Emőke J. E. "Non-Insulin Dependent Diabetes Mellitus among Aboriginal North Americans." *Annual Review of Anthropology* 23 (October 1994): 457–82. https://doi.org/10.1146/annurev.an.23.100194.002325.

Szathmáry, Emőke J. E., and R. E. Ferrell. "Glucose Level, Acculturation, and Glycosylated Hemoglobin: An Example of Biocultural Interaction." *Medical Anthropology Quarterly* 4, no. 3 (September 1990): 315–41. https://doi.org/10.1525/maq .1990.4.3.02a00040.

TallBear, Kim. "DNA, Blood, and Racializing the Tribe." *Wicazo Sa Review* 18, no. 1 (Spring 2003): 81–107. https://doi.org/10.1353/wic.2003.0008.

———. *Native American DNA: Tribal Belonging and the False Promise of Genetic Science*. Minneapolis: University of Minnesota Press, 2013.

Thompson, Samantha J., and Sandra M. Gifford. "Trying to Keep a Balance: The Meaning of Health and Diabetes in an Urban Aboriginal Community." *Social Science & Medicine* 51, no. 10 (November 2000): 1457–72. https://doi.org/10.1016/s0277 -9536(00)00046-0.

Thornton, Russell. *American Indian Holocaust and Survival: A Population History since 1492*. Norman: University of Oklahoma Press, 1987.

Thrush, Coll-Peter. *Native Seattle: Histories from the Crossing-Over Place*. Seattle: University of Washington Press, 2007.

Trafzer, Clifford E. *As Long as the Grass Shall Grow and Rivers Flow: A History of Native Americans*. Fort Worth TX: Harcourt College Publishers, 2000.

Trafzer, Clifford E., and Diane Weiner, eds. *Medicine Ways: Disease, Health, and Survival among Native Americans*. Walnut Creek CA: AltaMira Press, 2001.

Tsing, Anna Lowenhaupt. *Friction: An Ethnography of Global Connection*. Princeton: Princeton University Press, 2005.

Udler, Miriam S. "Type 2 Diabetes: Multiple Genes, Multiple Diseases." *Current Diabetes Reports* 19, no. 8 (August 2019): article 55 1–9. https://doi.org/10.1007/s11892 -019-1169-7.

United States Bureau of Indian Affairs. "A Brief History of Great Lakes Agency." Chicago: Newberry Library. Ayer Modern MS BIA Relocation, Box 1, Folder 4, 1975.

———. Indian Relocation Records, 1936–1975. Chicago: Newberry Library. Ayer Modern MS BIA Relocation, Boxes 1–3, 1975.

United States Census Bureau. "ACS Demographic and Housing Estimates 2006–2010, Chicago." Accessed October 20, 2012. http://factfinder2.census.gov/faces/tableservices/jsf/pages/productview.xhtml?src=bkmk.

Vaag, A. A., L. G. Grunnet, G. P. Arora, and C. Brøns. "The Thrifty Phenotype Hypothesis Revisited." *Diabetologia* 55, no. 8 (2012): 2085–88. https://doi.org/10.1007/s00125-012-2589-y.

Viruell-Fuentes, Edna A. "'My Heart Is Always There': The Transnational Practices of First-Generation Mexican Immigrant and Second-Generation Mexican American Women." *Identities: Global Studies in Culture and Power* 13, no. 3 (2006): 335–62. https://doi.org/10.1080/10702890600838076.

Vogel, Virgil J. "Indian Place Names in Illinois." *Journal of the Illinois State Historical Society (1908–1984)* 55, no. 1 (Spring 1962): 45–71.

Volscho, Thomas W. "Sterilization Racism and Pan-Ethnic Disparities of The Past Decade: The Continued Encroachment on Reproductive Rights." *Wicazo Sa Review* 25, no. 1 (Spring 2010): 17–31. https://doi.org/10.1353/wic.0.0053.

von Klein, Carl H. "The Medical Features of the Papyrus Ebers." *Journal of the American Medical Association* 45, no. 26 (December 1905): 1928–35. https://doi.org/10.1001/jama.1905.52510260014001e.

Watkins, Shanea, and James Sherk. "Who Serves in the U.S. Military? The Demographics of Enlisted Troops and Officers." Washington DC: Heritage Center for Data Analysis, 2008.

Weaver, Hilary N. "Indigenous Identity: What Is It, and Who Really Has It?" *American Indian Quarterly* 25, no. 2 (Spring 2001): 240–55. https://doi.org/10.1353/aiq.2001.0030.

Webster, A. "'To All the Former Cats and Stomps of the Navajo Nation': Performance, the Individual, and Cultural Poetic Traditions." *Language in Society* 37, no. 1 (February 2008): 61–89. https://doi.org/10.1017/S0047404508080032.

Weibel-Orlando, Joan. *Indian Country, L.A.: Maintaining Ethnic Community in Complex Society*. Urbana: University of Illinois Press, 1991.

Weiner, Diane. "Ethnogenetics: Interpreting Ideas about Diabetes and Inheritance." *American Indian Culture and Research Journal* 23, no. 3 (1999): 155–84. https://doi.org/10.17953/aicr.23.3.r322716j3l0r927h.

———. "Interpreting Ideas about Diabetes, Genetics, and Inheritance." In Trafzer and Weiner, *Medicine Ways*, 108–33.

Wendland, Claire L. *A Heart for the Work: Journeys through an African Medical School*. Chicago: University of Chicago Press, 2010.

West, Candace, and H. Zimmerman Don. "Doing Gender." *Gender and Society* 1, no. 2 (June 1987): 125–51. https://doi.org/10.1177/0891243287001002002.

West, Kelly M. "Diabetes in American Indian and Other Natives of the New World." *Diabetes* 23, no. 10 (October 1974): 841–55. https://doi.org/10.2337/diab.23.10.841.

Whitewater, Shannon, Kerstin M. Reinschmidt, Carmella Kahn, Agnes Attakai, and Nicolette I. Teufel-Shone. "Flexible Roles for American Indian Elders in Community-Based Participatory Research." *Preventing Chronic Disease* 13, no. E72 (June 2016): 1–6. https://doi.org/10.5888/pcd13.150575.

Whitmarsh, Ian. *Biomedical Ambiguity: Race, Asthma, and the Contested Meaning of Genetic Research in the Caribbean*. Ithaca NY: Cornell University Press, 2008.

Whyte, Susan Reynolds. "The Publics of the New Public Health: Life Conditions and 'Lifestyle Diseases' in Uganda." In *Making and Unmaking Public Health in Africa: Ethnographic and Historical Perspectives*, edited by Ruth J. Prince and Rebecca Marsland, 187–207. Athens: Ohio University Press, 2014.

Wiedman, Dennis. "Globalizing the Chronicities of Modernity: Diabetes and the Metabolic Syndrome." In *Chronic Conditions, Fluid States: Chronicity and the Anthropology of Illness*, edited by Lenore Manderson and Carolyn Smith-Morris, 38–53. New Brunswick: Rutgers University Press, 2010.

———. "Native American Embodiment of the Chronicities of Modernity: Reservation Food, Diabetes, and the Metabolic Syndrome among the Kiowa, Comanche, and Apache." *Medical Anthropology Quarterly* 26, no. 4 (December 2012): 595–612. https://doi.org/10.1111/maq.12009.

Wilkinson, Charles F., and Eric R. Briggs. "The Evolution of Termination Policy." *American Indian Law Review* 5, no. 1 (1977): 139–84. https://doi.org/10.2307/20068014.

Willard, William. "Indian Newspapers, or 'Say, Ain't You Some Kind of Indians?'" *Wicazo Sa Review* no. 10, no. 2 (Autumn 1994): 91–97. https://doi.org/10.2307/1409137.

Williams, Raymond. *Marxism and Literature*. Oxford: Oxford University Press, 1977.

Willis, Thomas, and Samuel Pordage. *Dr. Willis's Practice of Physick*. London: T. Dring, C. Harper, and J. Leigh, 1684.

Wilson, Natalia. "The Chicago Indian Village." In Straus, *Native Chicago*, 212–19.

Wilson, Robert, Carol Graham, Karmen G. Booth, and Dorothy Gohdes. "Community Approaches to Diabetes Prevention." In Joe and Young, *Diabetes as a Disease of Civilization*, 495–503.

Young, T Kue. "Diabetes among Canadian Indians and Inuit: An Epidemiological Overview." In Joe and Young, *Diabetes as a Disease of Civilization*, 21–40.

Zhao, Lu. "Self-Identification or Tribal Membership: Different Paths to Your Heritage." *Medill Reports*, Winter 2019. https://news.medill.northwestern.edu/chicago/self-identification-or-tribal-membership-different-paths-to-your-heritage/.

INDEX

Lightning Source UK Ltd.
Milton Keynes UK
UKHW011259290721
387960UK00001B/21